CBD

EVERY DAY

Also by Sandra Hinchliffe

Cannabis Spa at Home

High Tea

CBD
EVERY DAY

**HOW TO MAKE CANNABIS-INFUSED
MASSAGE OILS, BATH BOMBS, SALVES,
HERBAL REMEDIES, AND EDIBLES**

SANDRA HINCHLIFFE
Foreword by Dr. Stacey Kerr

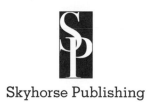

Skyhorse Publishing

Skyhorse Publishing books may be purchased in bulk at special discounts for sales promotion, corporate gifts, fund-raising, or educational purposes. Special editions can also be created to specifications. For details, contact the Special Sales Department, Skyhorse Publishing, 307 West 36th Street, 11th Floor, New York, NY 10018 or info@skyhorsepublishing.com.

Skyhorse® and Skyhorse Publishing® are registered trademarks of Skyhorse Publishing, Inc.®, a Delaware corporation.

Visit our website at www.skyhorsepublishing.com.

10 9 8 7 6 5

Library of Congress Cataloging-in-Publication Data is available on file.

Cover design by Qualcom
Cover photo credit: Sandra Hinchliffe

Print ISBN: 978-1-5107-4368-7
Ebook ISBN: 978-1-5107-4372-4

Printed in China

A special thanks to Jesse and Andrea Davis of Feather Canyon Farm Medical Collective, and Del Norte Sol~ personal care products. Jesse and Andrea Davis are local advocates for cannabis policy.

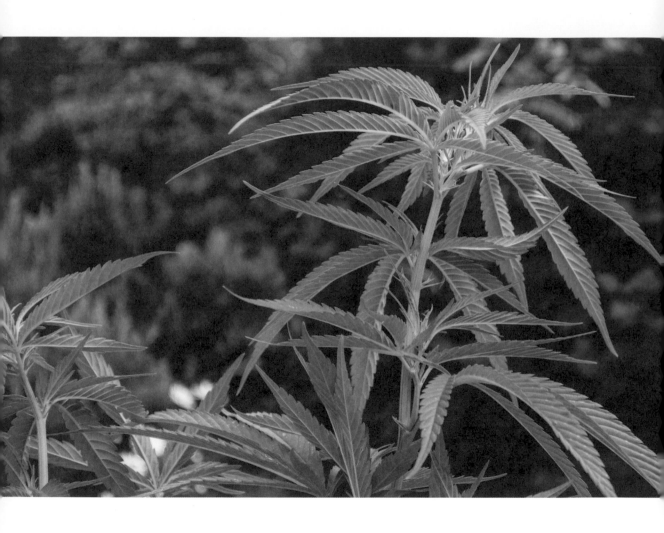

TABLE OF CONTENTS

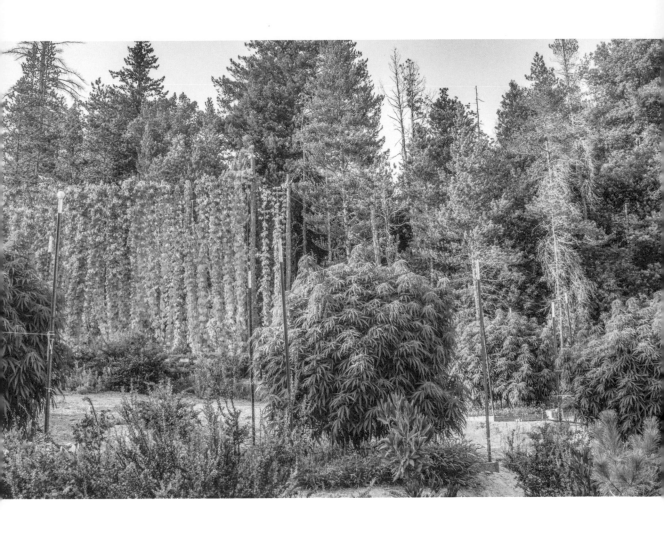

FOREWORD

Sandra has written a valuable book for anyone wishing to make their own products with cannabis flowers. As a family physician, I enjoy collaborating with patients willing to partner with me in maintaining their best health. Many of my patients here in Northern California use cannabis—I see the benefits daily—and with the discovery of CBD, even more people are finding uses for this lovely plant. I am convinced that cannabis used wisely can be a valuable ally, and Sandra's use of the whole plant to make so many helpful products is a real gift to us all.

With cannabis, we have a collaboration between herbal medicine and pharmaceuticals. The discovery of CBD and its uses has created a mass production of products for sale everywhere—medicines, beauty products, edibles, and many more. Fear of cannabis has lessened as we learn to use a more balanced ratio of cannabinoids, and with less fear of intoxication, these products are rapidly increasing in popularity. Some are being marketed as pharmaceuticals, but what about the personal relationship each of us has with the plant? Cannabis is a very individualized medicine—responding somewhat differently in everyone—and by making your own, you can tailor it to your specific needs. Those who make their own know exactly what is in it and where it all came from, a benefit many will find valuable. Some are always going to enjoy products bought at dispensaries, but many experienced as well as newly initiated users like to keep it more personal than that. Many would rather use a gentler herbal remedy before resorting to product made by pharmaceutical companies.

I have personally made medicine with cannabis flowers, and these recipes taught me even more than I ever imagined. The chapters on extraction methods are especially helpful. Who knew that putting an infusion in the freezer would prevent a grainy texture? Wonderful! Minty Chocolate Lip Balm sounds just too irresistible to pass up, and perhaps my chocolate mint growing in the garden can now be of some use in my kitchen. CBD is healing for skin problems, so the Whipped Chocolate Body Butter seems mighty tempting, with the lusciousness of chocolate combined with the healing qualities of CBD. It may seem complicated to make tinctures or spa products, but taken step-by-step your home kitchen, can turn into a personal pharmacy of helpful CBD products. From selecting the right product to the final creation, the information here is a treasure trove.

CBD and cannabis are going mainstream, but that does not mean we have to give up the personal aspects of this medicine. Whether your interest is in tinctures, topicals, edibles, or spa products, Sandra has you covered. All of these can support your efforts for best health. Specific ingredients, exact amounts, and detailed instructions are combined with luscious photos to give you all you need to create your own products with CBD. May this lovely book serve you well on your path to use this healing plant in a way that serves you best.

—Dr. Stacey Kerr, author of *Homebirth in the Hospital*
and contributing writer for Project CBD

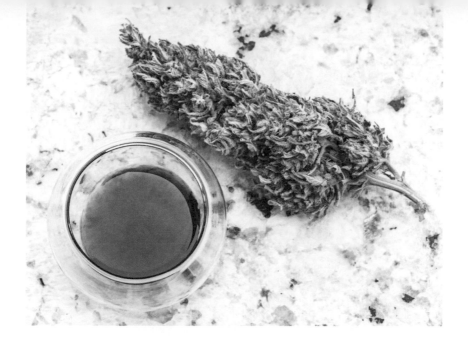

PREFACE

The recipes in this book are not intended for pregnant women, nursing mothers, or minors. The content of this book is solely the opinion and creation of the author and is not intended to be used as a substitute for a licensed MD or DO to advise about, diagnose, treat, cure, or prevent any disease or medical condition, and has not been approved by, or evaluated by the FDA. Nothing in this book is intended to encourage or promote illegal behavior and is not a substitute for advice from a licensed attorney.

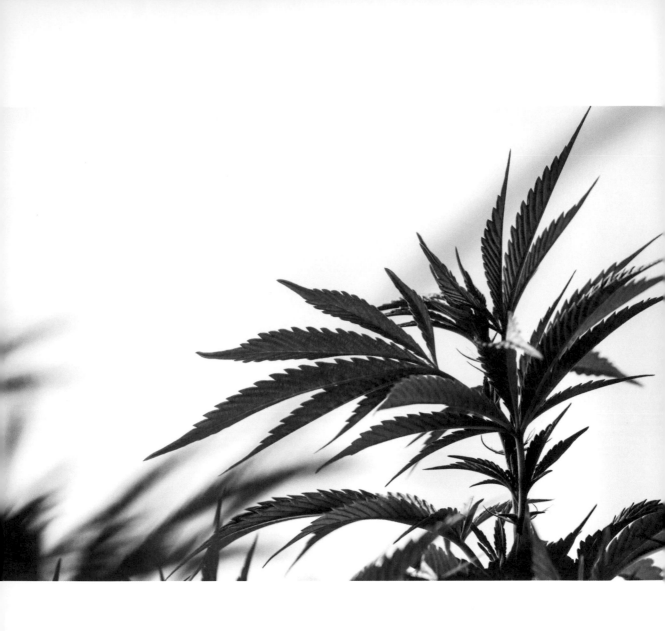

CHAPTER ONE

CBD IS CANNABIS

CBD: Cannabidiol Defined

CBD (Cannabidiol) is a *cannabinoid* occurring naturally in the cannabis plant in varying percentages. More than 60 different types of cannabinoids have been described in scientific literature, with CBD occurring in the most concentrated amounts, after THC (Tetrahydrocannabinol).[1] CBD was first analyzed and described in depth by Dr. Raphael Mechoulam in 1963.[2]

It should be noted here that CBD doesn't start out as CBD in raw cannabis plant material. CBD begins as CBDA (Cannabidiolic acid) and becomes CBD through the process of decarboxylation in which carbon atoms are dropped from the original CBDA molecule over time, or through the application of heat, or with both heat and time.

CBD is specific to the *Cannabis sativa* plant and does not occur in any other plant. However, similar cannabinoid-like chemistry can be found throughout the plant kingdom, such as the terpene beta-caryophyllene in

---

1 "Chemistry and Analysis of Phytocannabinoids and Other Cannabis Constituents," *Medical Genomics*, Rudolf Brenneisen, https://www.medicinalgenomics.com/wp-content/uploads/2011/12/Chemical-constituents-of-cannabis.pdf.
2 "Hashish. I. The structure of cannabidiol," *Tetrahedron* 19: 2073–2078, R. Mechoulam and Y. Shvo. (1963) https://www.ncbi.nlm.nih.gov/pubmed/5879214.

black pepper, cloves, and carnations, which has affinity for CB2 receptors.[3] More studies are needed to understand the relationship of cannabinoids like CBD and cannabinoid-like substances in other plants to the endocannabinoid system as well as their effects and usefulness for humans and animals.

CBD has become one of the most talked about and promising plant medicines of the twenty-first century. Apart from the documented medicinal effects of CBD,[4] many people are interested in this cannabinoid simply for the gentle, sober relief and relaxation effects that they have experienced while consuming CBD-rich cannabis plants and products.

Most people who consume CBD plants and products report that there is no psychoactive "high" from CBD. When compared to THC, the psychoactive effects and the health concerns for which CBD is therapeutic are not completely understood by scientists at the time of publication of this book.[5] Your experience with CBD will depend on many factors, so it is important to embark on this exploration with both an open mind and skepticism.

Cannabis sativa: CBD-Rich Cannabis Strains and Hemp

CBD comes from the *Cannabis sativa* plant and cannot be divorced from this original source. *Cannabis sativa* has many different variations, and not all of these contain significant amounts of CBD. Prior to the gradual

---

3   "The cannabinoid CB2 receptor-selective phytocannabinoid beta-caryophyllene exerts analgesic effects in mouse models of inflammatory and neuropathic pain," *European Neuropsychopharmacology*, A.-L. Klauke et al. Volume 24, Issue 4, 608–620 https://www.europeanneuropsychopharmacology.com/article/S0924-977X(13)00302-7/fulltext.

4   EPIDIOLEX (cannabidiol) oral solution—FDA approved epilepsy treatment drug, package insert and prescribing information https://www.accessdata.fda.gov/drugsatfda_docs/label/2018/210365lbl.pdf.

5   "Cannabidiol: State of the art and new challenges for therapeutic applications," *Pharmacology & Therapeutics*, S. Pisanti et al. 175: 133–150. https://www.ncbi.nlm.nih.gov/pubmed/28232276.

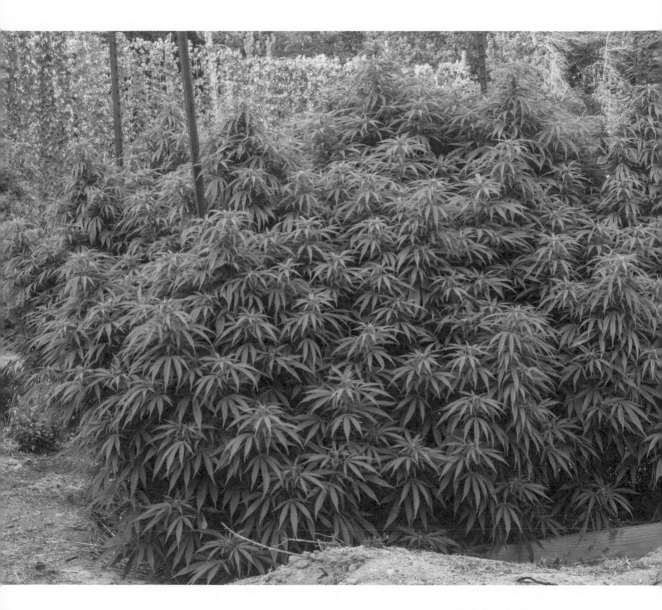

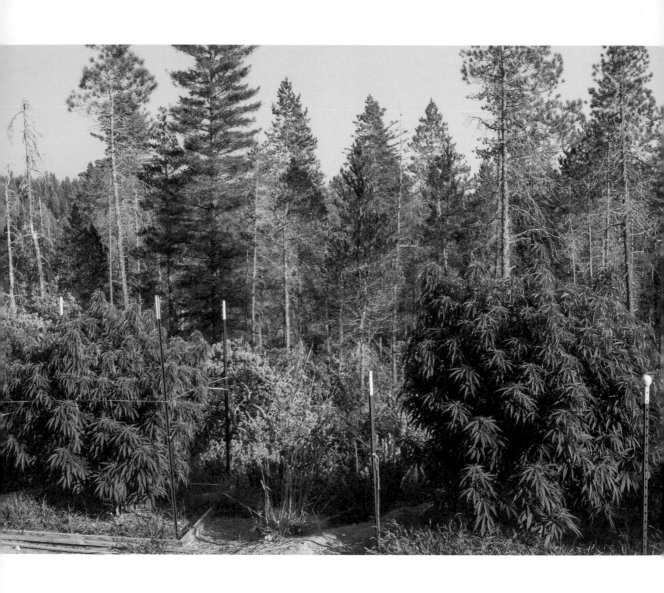

ending of cannabis prohibition in many locales, CBD was practically eliminated from the commercial black market to maximize profitability of the psychoactive cannabinoid content of the plants through selective breeding, according to many of the black-market growers I have spoken with throughout the years. The reason CBD is now widely accessible is most assuredly due to the change in social perceptions of this once-outlawed plant and the legalization of this plant in many locales. Without cannabis legalization, CBD would be difficult to acquire—and there would be no testing to ensure that consumers receive the product they are paying for.

In the process of developing my recipes for this book, I spent much of my time talking to CBD farmers and exploring their lush farms. I am forever grateful to my friends at Feather Canyon Farms in Del Norte County, California, for introducing me to some of the most impressive plants I've ever seen in my life. Beforehand, my experience with these plants had been limited to small indoor grows and the product offerings of our legal cannabis dispensaries.

One of the things I learned from the CBD farmers is that CBD can be an unstable and fleeting trait in cannabis plants. CBD production doesn't just depend on the genetics of a plant, but the methods of growing, and what is also recognized in grape and wine production as the terroir. New strains of CBD-rich cannabis are being developed for the legal market all the time. I haven't been able to try them all, but I've had the privilege of trying some of the most well-known strains, such as Harlequin, Harle-Tsu, ACDC, Cannatonic, Charlotte's Web, Sour Tsunami, and a rare crop of Golden Goat, which expressed more than 8% CBD. This list is by no means complete in terms of CBD-rich cannabis strains available.

Hemp, the low-to-no THC variety of *Cannabis sativa* grown for the oilseed and fiber it produces, can also produce CBD in varying amounts. Both wild hemp and cultivated hemp can produce CBD in their resins. No matter what variety of *Cannabis sativa* produces CBD, the molecule is always the same.

Farmers, Plants, and Test Results over Brands: How To Select CBD Products

I believe that quality, whole-plant infusions and extractions matter. Epidiolex, the FDA-approved drug, is a whole-plant extract of CBD, purified, standardized, and manufactured for consistency. It's rare as far as pharmaceuticals go; GW Pharma grows and processes their own cannabis to make therapeutic pharmaceuticals.[6] Whether you are in need of a pharmaceutical treatment or are using CBD as a home remedy or for pleasure, you should be using whole-plant infusions and extractions. The cannabis farmers I spoke with have expressed a similar belief.

In my opinion, everything great about CBD begins and ends with the farmers who grow the plants. And since this recipe book is all about CBD as a home remedy or for pleasure, telling the story of the farmers I have met and bringing their farms to you through the stories, pictures, and recipes here is my gift to you; this is the essence of what it means to select and consume quality CBD-rich cannabis plant products.

I am often asked about which brands of CBD are the best and which products to choose. But the truth is that when it comes to CBD, brands

---

6 Greenwich Biosciences Announces FDA Approval of EPIDIOLEX® (cannabidiol) Oral Solution—the First Plant-derived Cannabinoid Prescription Medicine, Press Release, June 25, 2018. https://www.greenwichbiosciences.com/about-us/news/green wich-biosciences-announces-fda-approval-epidiolex%C2%AE-cannabidiol-oral -solution-%E2%80%93.

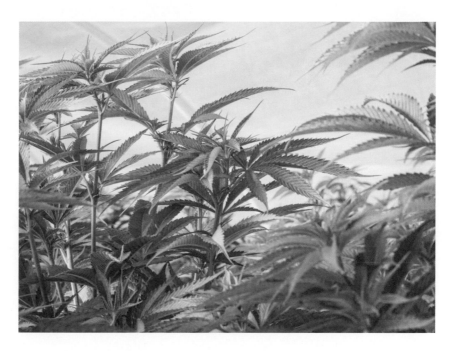

do not matter. Farms and plants matter. Selecting quality CBD-rich cannabis plant products begins with the farm they are grown on. Before you purchase any CBD product, know the farm and farmer. This is an easy task in most of our state-legal cannabis dispensaries, as this information will be readily available and even used as a marketing tool. This information is harder to find if you are purchasing CBD products from the over-the-counter herbal supplement market.

CBD products sold over the counter in the mainstream herbal supplement market do not have the oversight and regulated testing that most of our state-legal dispensary systems have. If you choose to purchase CBD products in the herbal supplement market, you must rely on the information they provide to you in terms of acquisition of plant material and test results. You must also be aware that there is controversy (both legal and

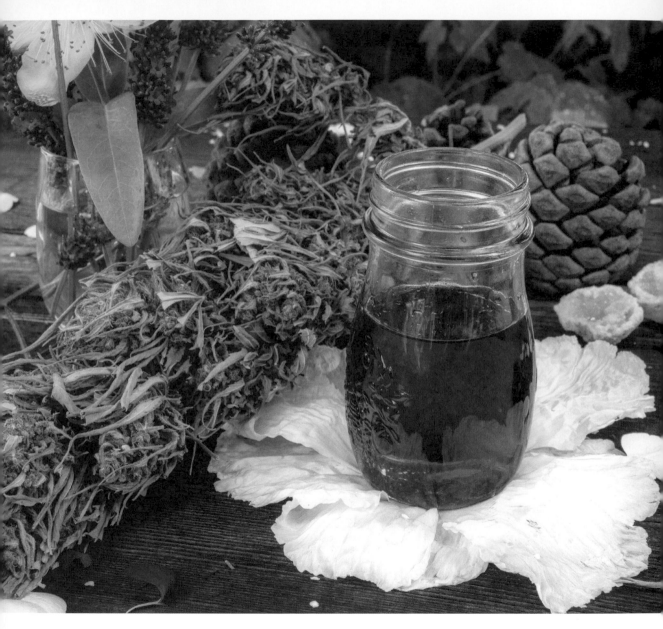

scientific) surrounding the purchase of CBD products over the counter through the mainstream herbal supplement marketplace.

Test results matter. The herbal supplement marketplace is largely unregulated and a bit like the Wild West. An exposé in the *New York Times* in 2013 detailed some very disturbing problems with the herbal supplement marketplace and the fact that consumers often do not receive the products they are paying for.[7] As well, CBD supplement merchants in the over-the-counter herbal supplement market have been cited by the FDA for many violations around the labeling and distribution of their products.[8]

Certainly, I am not saying that all herbal supplement products are bad. What I am saying is that it is a wise decision as a consumer to seek out information and verify it if you are purchasing supplement products of any kind. And you should also be aware that not all locales will regard the purchase of CBD products as a legal activity.

The functionality of this book is to show you how to seek, find, and enjoy CBD-rich cannabis. Facts and aesthetics both matter if what you seek is a quality product and a satisfying experience.

In the recipes that follow, the focus is on whole-plant CBD-rich cannabis extractions and infusions, as these high-quality, artisanal, and farmer-centric whole plants and whole-plant resins will unfold themselves with fragrant and delicious complexity in your kitchen. My wish is for you to enjoy and benefit from everything CBD-rich cannabis offers without missing anything.

---

7   "Herbal Supplements Are Often Not What They Seem," *New York Times*, A. O'Connor, November 3, 2013, https://www.nytimes.com/2013/11/05/science/herbal-supplements-are-often-not-what-they-seem.html.

8   Warning Letters and Test Results for Cannabidiol-Related Products, FDA.gov https://www.fda.gov/newsevents/publichealthfocus/ucm484109.htm.

CBD to THC Ratio Selection and Dosing

Selection and dosage amount of CBD or CBD:THC is a very individual process and an ideal dosage that works as a one-size-fits-all amount does not exist. If you have concerns about what is best for you, this is something you should discuss with your personal physician. There are also MDs and DOs who specialize in cannabis therapeutics who can guide you based on your current health situation. If you are considering CBD for therapeutic medicinal purposes, it's a good idea to consult with a physician who has knowledge and experience in this area before you begin.

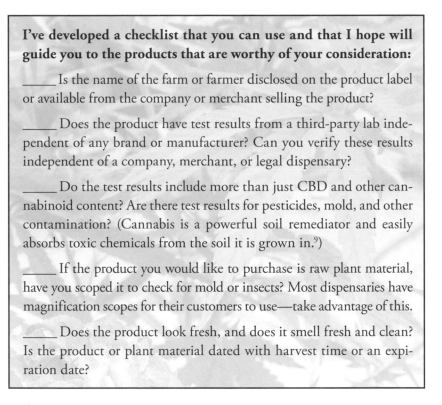

I've developed a checklist that you can use and that I hope will guide you to the products that are worthy of your consideration:

_____ Is the name of the farm or farmer disclosed on the product label or available from the company or merchant selling the product?

_____ Does the product have test results from a third-party lab independent of any brand or manufacturer? Can you verify these results independent of a company, merchant, or legal dispensary?

_____ Do the test results include more than just CBD and other cannabinoid content? Are there test results for pesticides, mold, and other contamination? (Cannabis is a powerful soil remediator and easily absorbs toxic chemicals from the soil it is grown in.[9])

_____ If the product you would like to purchase is raw plant material, have you scoped it to check for mold or insects? Most dispensaries have magnification scopes for their customers to use—take advantage of this.

_____ Does the product look fresh, and does it smell fresh and clean? Is the product or plant material dated with harvest time or an expiration date?

Just because a CBD-rich product has some THC in it does not mean that you will experience the "high" associated with cannabis. Many of the highest quality products and whole-plant preparations will contain small amounts of THC at 1% or greater. In fact, it is this "entourage effect" of all the whole-plant constituents—the cannabinoids and terpenes—that create the highest quality and most effective CBD products. This effect has been discussed by researchers such as Dr. Sanjay Gupta on nationwide platforms such as CNN.

In my experience preparing CBD-rich recipes for others, most adults will not experience psychoactive effects at a 1% THC level or less, especially if the CBD levels are much higher than that. If I were introducing cannabis to an elderly person, or someone who has never tried cannabis, I would probably serve them a remedy, beverage, or edible with 10mg to 25mg of CBD and 1mg to 2mg THC. If they are interested in experiencing a hint of the euphoric effects of THC in a very gentle manner, I'd use the 2mg. In my experience serving others, noticeable and pleasant effects with CBD really start at around a 10mg dose. Because CBD is not psychoactive the way THC is, even higher doses up to 50mg or more are fine. CBD may cause some drowsiness in higher doses, so keep this in mind.

Never drive or operate machinery while under the influence of anything. Remember that this is for relief, relaxation, recreation, and enlightenment—not for drive time!

In our legal-state dispensaries, you will often find CBD cannabis products labeled with their ratios as well as milligram content or percentage of cannabinoids. These ratios will vary, with some of the highest CBD at 30:1 CBD to THC. A 30:1 ratio will have no intoxicating or noticeable

---

9 "Industrial hemp (Cannabis sativa L.) growing on heavy metal contaminated soil: fibre quality and phytoremediation potential," *Industrial Crops and Products,* Volume 16, Issue 1, July 2002, pages 33–42, P. Lingera, J. Müssig, H. Fischer, J. Koberta. https://www.sciencedirect.com/science/article/pii/S0926669002000055.

psychoactivity. You will encounter labels with lower ratios such as 10:2, or 5:2, or 3:1. Just because the ratio is lower does not mean there will be intoxicating effects. These ratios serve as a guideline for you; when you find a ratio you enjoy, this is something you can use for further reference whether you intend to purchase CBD plant material or product or if you later choose to grow your own.

Avoiding the psychoactive effects that can be caused by THC can be accomplished by calculating the percentages of each cannabinoid as exact milligram dosages. Keep in mind that CBD does attenuate the effects of THC and will create a gentler high. If you choose to consume higher doses of THC, match that with a higher dose of CBD. CBD is also useful for someone who is uncomfortable with the effects of THC, as it will lessen anxiety.

Here is an example of how to calculate the milligram dosage in a raw cannabis plant product, whole plant, or resin where the percentage of cannabinoids are known: 1 gram of CBD-rich cannabis flower or plant material, 10% CBD and 1% THC.

$$1 \text{ gram} = 1000 \text{ milligrams}$$
$$1000\text{mg} \times .10 = 100\text{mg CBD}$$
$$1000\text{mg} \times .01 = 10\text{mg THC}$$

The 1 gram of the CBD-rich whole cannabis plant material you have selected can be portioned into 10 servings with 10mg of CBD and 1mg THC per serving. (Approximately! This will depend on the actual amounts obtained through the decarboxylation process and may be less but will not be more if the percentages of cannabinoids provided to you are correct.)

CBD resins such as sifted hash or resin oil will follow the same calculation process but will be more concentrated in cannabinoids than whole-plant material. Here is an example for either of these, assuming an example of 50% CBD and 5% THC:

1 gram of raw sifted hash or resin oil = 1000 milligrams

1000mg x .50 = 500mg CBD

1000mg x .05 = 50mg THC

If this is portioned into 20 servings, each serving should contain 25mg CBD and 2.5mg THC. (Again, approximately! This will depend on the actual amounts obtained through the decarboxylation process and may be less but will not be more if the percentages of cannabinoids provided to you are correct.)

CBD resin oils that are decarboxylated and labeled with their exact milligram dosage for both CBD and THC are available at most legal state dispensaries. This is a good product for beginners who are just starting their journey! This product can be incorporated into any of the recipes in this book and can be diluted into carrier fats and used in recipes as described in chapter 2.

Relief, Relaxation, Recreation, and Enlightenment— Without the High

My own journey with the cannabis plant has been an interesting one. As I get older, I find that cannabis affects me differently than it did even a decade ago. I find myself gravitating more toward topical and spa products and to CBD-rich preparations. I find that gentle euphoria, with lots of pain and inflammation relief, is really the sweet spot for me. I have a difficult time enjoying CBD that has been completely divorced from THC, however. Even a small amount of THC, 1mg or so, increases the relief and relaxation I experience with CBD. For me, that delightful, sweet-spot dose looks more like 25mg CBD and 5mg THC, which has all the benefits of CBD with gentle and mild euphoria. This is why I enjoy and advocate for whole-plant CBD preparations.

CBD-rich cannabis makes it possible for you to enjoy cannabis without any high or euphoric effect at all, if this is what you desire. The CBD-rich

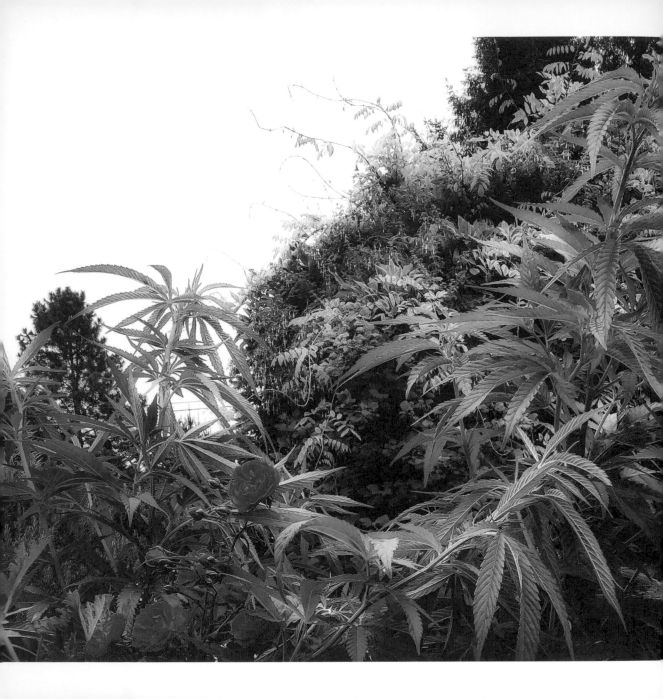

cannabis experience can be as sober as you would like it to be. We have a saying here in California: the cannabis dispensary is not just for people who want to get high! CBD products are some of the most in-demand products available at our legal dispensaries. Everyone is different, and older people as well as new consumers, especially, will find that their experience will vary, so it is best to begin with lower dosages of both CBD and THC and wait an hour or two before consuming more.

In the recipes that follow, you will be able to create your own relief, relaxation, recreation, and enlightenment with CBD-rich plants and products in the dosage levels and forms of consumption that are the most satisfying for you.

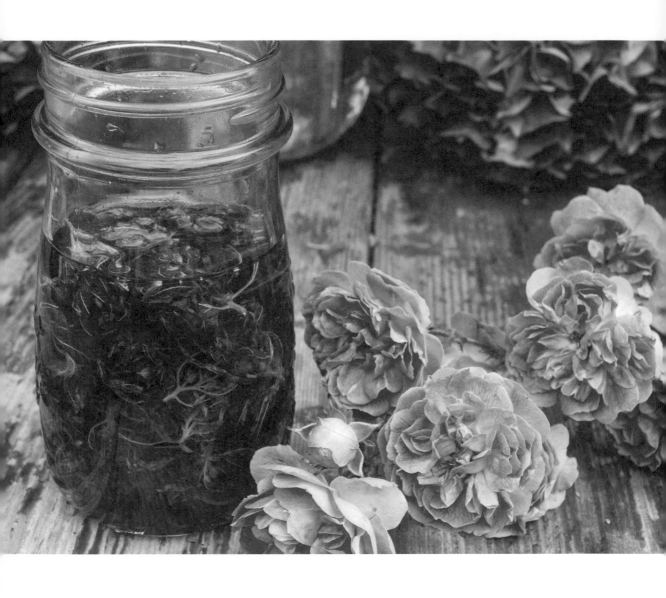

CHAPTER TWO

CBD AND CBDA EXTRACTION METHODS AND RECIPES

Forms of CBD

You will encounter whole-plant CBD in the following forms: whole-plant material, sifted hash, resin oil, or as a commercially prepared product already diluted in a carrier oil or other culinary solvent.

Whole-plant material: This is just what you would expect—a whole plant consisting of mostly flowers and some leaf. Shake, otherwise known as trimmed leaf, is also another form of whole-plant material.

Sifted hash: This is produced by separating the trichomes from the plant material through various processes, including hand rubbing, kief shaking, and ice-water hash processing methods. Sifted hash products are whole-plant cannabis concentrates.

Resin oil: This is produced by processing whole-plant material in culinary ethyl alcohol or by pressing the resins from the flowers using heat or pressure. Some of the names of this oil you may encounter are: RSHO, RSO, full-extract cannabis oil, rosin, or live resin. If you have a commercially prepared product that is already in carrier oil or culinary solvent appropriate for the recipe, you can use that directly in the recipe without further preparation, unless you would like to dilute it further.

CBD Farmer's Oil Recipe with Whole Flowers

The CBD oil depicted in the photo for this recipe is very special to me. When one considers flavors, textures, freshness, effects, and fragrances as the starting point of evaluating a quality CBD oil product, this recipe will produce a gourmet oil extraction that will impress even the most experienced connoisseur.

Farmers know best. And this oil recipe was given to me by one of the most hardworking and knowledgeable CBD farmers I have met, Mr. Jesse Davis of Feather Canyon Farms in Del Norte County, California.

I experienced many pleasant surprises while sampling this oil at home, and the process of making it was even more surprising. Rich in both CBD and the natural terpenes of the Harle-Tsu CBD-rich cannabis plant, this oil is a gorgeous emerald color with a sublime minty and herbaceous flavor that I have never experienced with a CBD oil previously. This oil was completely non-intoxicating, but it was very pleasant and relaxing.

This oil, processed in MCT oil (fractionated coconut oil) at a low temperature for 24 hours, produced a CBD oil product that has lab tested at 10mg CBD and less than 1mg THC per 1ml dose. How low was that temperature? 175°F (80°C)—a temperature much lower than what is typically expected for a complete decarboxylation. What made the difference? The slow processing of this oil over a 24-hour period. Decarboxylation takes place with temperature, time, or in this case, both time and temperature.

I am satisfied that the flavor profile of this oil was only possible due to the careful, low-temperature processing technique that retained the majority of naturally occurring terpenes in the whole cannabis flowers from the CBD-rich Harle-Tsu cannabis strain grown in the mountain region of Del Norte County. Flower quality really does matter when it comes to producing an exquisite CBD oil such as this one.

This makes approximately 10 oz (296ml) of CBD oil, but you can increase or decrease the amount of oil or flowers depending on the CBD concentration you desire.

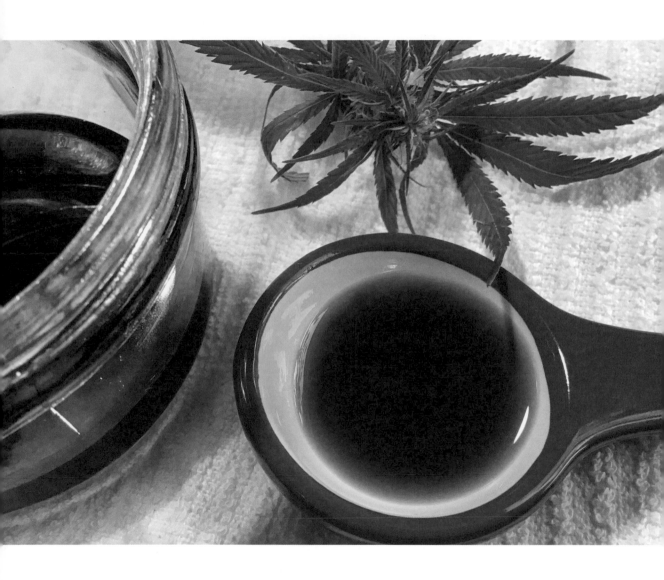

CBD and CBDA Extraction Methods and Recipes   19

1. This recipe requires a slow cooker with a low heat setting to process this oil correctly. Add the chopped cannabis to the slow cooker.
2. Pour the oil over the cannabis, making sure that all the flower material is covered. If you need to add a little extra oil to cover the flowers, you should do so at this time. Cover the slow cooker and set to the low or low cook setting (depending on your model).
3. Within at least 3 hours, your slow cooker should reach the final processing temperature of about 175°F (80°C). Use a candy thermometer to verify the temperature and adjust if necessary. Stir the oil and plant material at this time and cover the slow cooker once again.
4. Every few hours, stir the oil and flower material to evenly distribute the infusion throughout the process. Do not stir frequently, as this will allow more of the volatile terpenes to escape into the air. To preserve as many of the volatile constituents as possible, such as terpenes, leave the lid on the pot throughout the entire process. This can be left to process overnight without stirring.
5. After the 24-hour period is over, cool the oil by unplugging the slow cooker and allowing the materials to remain in the pot and the oil to cool to room temperature a few more hours.
6. Strain the oil from the plant material through cheesecloth and into a clean glass jar. The oil is now ready to use by itself in measured doses or in any recipe. Store in a cool, dark, and dry area. Use within 6 months for freshest flavor.

10 oz (296ml) MCT oil or more (otherwise known as liquid fractionated coconut oil)

1 oz (28g) or more whole CBD-rich, low-or-no-THC cannabis flowers, cured, dried, and chopped

Slow cooker

CBD Infusion Recipe with Olive Oil, Camellia Seed Oil, Sunflower Seed Oil, and Rice Bran Oil

I have long been an advocate of cannabis-infused oils that are high in oleic acid. Particularly, I love olive oil, as it is high in oleic acid, but it's also a simple ingredient that is easy to obtain at the local supermarket. Olive oil

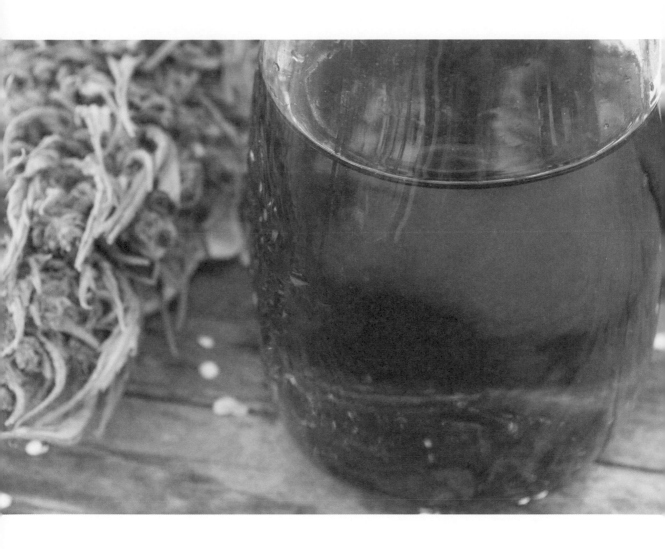

has also been demonstrated to be a superior extractor of cannabinoids and other cannabis constituents even when stacked up against naphtha and ethanol![10] You should feel confident that your olive oil infusions will be high quality when performed correctly.

You may be interested in experimenting with other oils. Next to olive oil, camellia seed oil (the seed oil of the tea plant, not to be confused with tea tree oil!) really shines in anything topical, from beauty creams to salves. It has almost no fragrance of its own, unlike olive oil. It also absorbs into the skin more quickly than any of the other oils I have listed here.

Sunflower seed oil is similar to olive oil and absorbs into the skin about as quickly. Rice bran oil, while it is high in oleic acid, tends to be less absorbent than the other oils in this group. I like rice bran oil for mature skin or for massage.

Quality matters when it comes to olive oil, or any oil for that matter. Check for purity and expiration dates to obtain the best results with your CBD infusions.

Whole-Plant CBD Infusion with Flower/Leaf or Sifted Hashes

To retain as much of the natural terpene content as possible, this method, which uses standard canning jars like mason jars, and a canning bath or stockpot with boiling water, prevents escape of any of the delicate volatile oils during the decarboxylation process. Using flower and leaf will retain

---

10 "Cannabis Oil: chemical evaluation of an upcoming cannabis-based medicine" *IACM Journal,* Cannabinoids 2013;1(1):1–11, Luigi L. Romano, Arno Hazekamp Department of Pharmacy, University of Siena, Italy Plant Metabolomics group, Institute of Biology, Leiden University, The Netherlands. http://www.cannabis-med.org/data/pdf/en_2013_01_1.pdf.

full cannabis fragrances and flavors. Using a sifted hashish will produce a CBD oil infusion with less fragrance. Both are whole-plant infusions, but one or the other may be useful for different things such as spa products like lotions or creams where the fragrance of cannabis may not be desirable.

CBD-rich cannabis flowers and trim or sifted hashish, chopped

One of the oils in this group: olive, camellia, sunflower, rice bran

1 pint (500ml) canning jar and lid, or larger, depending on how much oil you would like to make

A canning bath or a stockpot filled with water

1. Calculate the approximate dosage amounts that you desire. Making this oil very concentrated will enable you to use it in other recipes in smaller amounts. This is a base CBD oil that can be used in any of your own recipes after you make it.
2. In a clean glass canning jar, add the cannabis plant material and pour the oil over it at least 1 inch (2.5cm) above the plant material or more. The jar should have at least 2 inches (5cm) of headspace at the very top, no matter how much cannabis or oil you decide to use. Screw the lid on tightly.
3. Fill the canning bath or stockpot with water and place the jar with the oil and cannabis into the water. Turn the heat to medium-high and bring to a boil with the jar in the water. Process for 3 to 4 hours, adding more water to the canning bath or stockpot as needed. Do not allow this to boil dry as it will explode the canning jar.
4. Remove the jar from the canning bath or stockpot and allow it to completely cool on the counter. You will notice that the canning jar has "sealed" itself once the jar is cool, so take care in opening the jar so as not to spill the oil.
5. Filter the oil through a cheesecloth into another clean glass jar. Squeeze out as much of the oil as possible. Affix the lid and store in a cool and dark place for up to 6 months for best flavor and effects.

Whole-Plant CBD Infusion with Full Extract, RSO, or Resins

Full-extract oil or resins will come as either CBDA (not decarboxylated) or as CBD (already decarboxylated). If you need to decarboxylate to obtain CBD, simply follow the recipe steps for the whole plant and sifted hash decarboxylation process and then add oil or resin to one of the carrier oils listed here in the calculated serving sizes you desire.

If you prefer CBDA, gently and quickly melt the oil or resin into the carrier oil on low heat until it is fully combined, and transfer to a clean jar immediately. Storing this in a cool place like the refrigerator and using within 3 months will ensure greater amounts of CBDA are retained.

CBD Infusion Recipe with Coconut Oil, Cacao Butter, and Murumuru Butter

Solid fats in this group can undergo the same infusion process with CBD-rich cannabis as liquid fats can, but you do have to make a few tweaks. For this group of fats, infusion using a slow cooker or double boiler will probably be easier than using the canning jar and canning bath/stockpot method, but to fully retain terpenes and all of the chemical constituents of whole-plant infusions, using the canning jar method will work best. Terpenes tend to release into the air without a tight seal like those offered by canning jars. But a slow cooker or double boiler will still process a lovely infused oil, so I will leave this up to you and give instruction here for all these methods.

CBD-rich cannabis flowers and trim or sifted hashish, chopped
One of the oils in this group: coconut, cacao butter, murumuru butter
A metal strainer and cheesecloth
1 pint (500ml) canning jar and lid, or larger, depending on how much oil you would like to make
A canning bath or a stockpot filled with water
OR
A slow cooker or lidded double boiler (no canning jar necessary)

Instructions for processing in a canning jar and canning bath or stockpot:

1. Calculate the approximate dosage amounts that you desire. Making this oil very concentrated will enable you to use it in other recipes in smaller amounts. This is a base CBD oil that can be used in any of your own recipes after you make it.
2. Gently melt the solid fat you have chosen on low heat first. In a clean glass canning jar, add the cannabis plant material and pour the melted oil over it at least 1 inch (2.5cm) above the plant material or more. The jar should have at least 2 inches (5cm) of headspace at the very top, no matter how much cannabis or oil you decide to use. Screw the lid on tightly.
3. Fill the canning bath or stockpot water and place the jar with the oil and cannabis into the water. Turn on the heat to medium-high and bring to a boil with the jar in the water. Process for 3 to 4 hours, adding more water to the canning bath or stockpot as needed. Do not allow this to boil dry, as it will explode the canning jar.

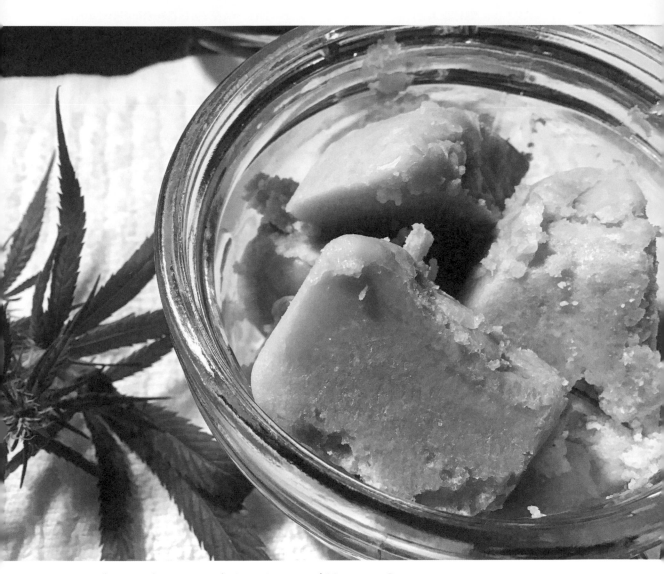

CBD Infusion with Coconut Oil, Cacao Butter, and Murumuru Butter

4. Remove the jar from the canning bath or stockpot and allow it to cool just enough that you can safely handle the jar. Keep in mind that these fats will turn solid again rather quickly, and you want to filter this oil from the plant material before it starts to solidify. If the canning jar has "sealed" itself, take care in opening the jar so as not to spill the oil. Potholders and gloves are useful in decanting the oil from the jar to prevent burns and spills!

5. Working quickly so that the oil does not solidify, filter the oil through a cheesecloth into another clean glass jar. Squeeze out as much of the oil as possible.

6. Allow the jar to cool for 15 to 20 minutes on the counter. Affix the lid, then transfer to the freezer to solidify it quickly. This will prevent a grainy texture from forming in the hardened oil. Store in a cool and dark place for up to 6 months for best flavor and effects.

Instructions for processing in a slow cooker or double boiler:

1. Melt the fat in the slow cooker or double boiler. Add the chopped cannabis or sifted hashish, making sure that it is completely covered in oil.

2. Put on the lid and process on high for 3 hours in the slow cooker or simmer in the double boiler on medium to medium-high for the same amount of time. To preserve as many of the volatile constituents as possible, such as terpenes, leave the lid on the pot throughout the entire process.

3. After processing, turn off the slow cooker or remove the processing pan from the double boiler. Allow the oil to briefly cool, covered, for only 10 minutes or so, ensuring that the fats do not solidify.

4. Line a strainer with cheesecloth and ladle the oil through the strainer into a clean glass heat-resistant jar. Work quickly so that the oil does not solidify but also carefully as the oil will be hot.

5. Allow the jar to cool for 15 to 20 minutes on the counter. Affix the lid then transfer to the freezer to solidify it quickly. This will prevent

a grainy texture from forming in the hardened oil. Store in a cool and dark place for up to 6 months for best flavor and effects.

Alternatively, you may also infuse CBD into one of these solid fats using the CBD Farmer's Oil recipe in this chapter and process using a slow cooker on low heat for 24 hours. This makes a fine infusion! You will need to melt the solid fat first, as described here, before adding it to the crockpot with the cannabis flowers as described in the CBD Farmer's Oil recipe.

CBD and CBDA Tincture Recipe

Making CBD-infused tinctures is an easy way to prepare CBD-rich cannabis for use in many herbal remedies. A good-quality tincture requires some very powerful alcohol; grain or any culinary-grade alcohol (150-proof or more) is required—anything less will be disappointing. Higher proofs are always better for creating tinctures, so if these higher-proof alcohols are available where you live, you will obtain the best results by using them. While these are culinary-grade, they are also extremely flammable, and you should not work with them around any open flame or spark. I always tincture with my kitchen window open and all appliances, except for the refrigerator, turned off.

Choose the whole-plant form that will work best for your needs. Whole flowers and leaves will lend their chlorophyll to the tincture and make it a lovely emerald color just like whole-plant oil infusions. Sifted hashish will have less or no chlorophyll. Full-extract or RSO will contain chlorophyll, similar to the flower and leaf tincture. Raw resins and rosin will be similar to sifted hashish. Chlorophyll has some of its own benefits as an antioxidant, and I prefer tinctures with it.

Once you have chosen the form of CBD-rich cannabis you would like to use in your tincture, you will want to make this as concentrated as possible so that it can serve as a base tincture for other recipes. You may also enjoy it on its own and make it as concentrated or mild as you desire.

If you are using flowers, leaves, or sifted hashish, there is a good chance that they are not decarboxylated, which is a step you need to perform before you make the tincture. If the plant material you have chosen is already decarboxylated, or if you desire to tincture mostly CBDA, you may move forward with the tincturing part of the recipe, skipping the decarboxylation step.

You will hear a lot of different opinions about the exact temperature to decarboxylate CBDA into CBD! In some experiments, I have found

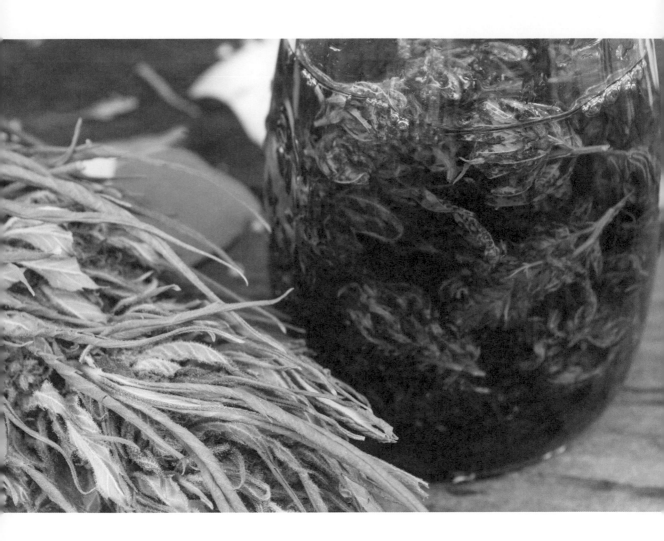

that 275° F (135° C) for 60 minutes has produced tinctures that are rich in CBD. I most often decarb for 90 minutes, and this produces the best tincture in my experience. Decarboxylating your cannabis material longer than 90 minutes at that temperature may impart undesirable flavors, so it's best to use this temperature (275° F) and time (90 minutes) for the best flavors in my experience.

Decarboxylation Process

The amount and form of CBD-rich cannabis that you desire, to be processed in a glass or silicone baking dish with a lid.

1. Preheat the oven to 275° F (135° C).
2. Place whatever form of cannabis you have selected into a glass or silicone baking dish with a lid. There is no need to chop the plant material for this process.
3. Process in the oven for 90 minutes, covered with a lid that fits well to prevent as much of the terpene content from escaping as possible. Remove from the oven and allow to cool on the counter before coarsely chopping to perform the tincture process if you are using flowers, leaves, or large chunks of hashish material.

CBD Tincturing

Any decarboxylated CBD-rich cannabis plant material (flowers and leaves, sifted hashish, resin oil, etc.)
150-proof or higher culinary-grade alcohol
1 glass canning jar with sealable lid
Large pot to hold warm water
Funnel lined with cheesecloth
Glass tincture bottles with bulb dropper caps

1. Calculate the final concentration of CBD, per serving, number of servings, and the serving size that you desire. The typical serving size of a dropperful is ¼ teaspoon to ⅔ teaspoon (1ml to 3ml). Since you will be working with high-proof alcohol, creating serving sizes that are no greater than 1 teaspoon (5ml), which is high in CBD concentration, is the best for ensuring alcohol consumption is negligible when using tinctures orally.
2. Coarsely chop the decarboxylated plant material and break up any hard hashish or resins. Put the plant material into the glass canning jar. Based on the calculations you have made, add the amount of alcohol needed to create your desired servings. Alcohol should always

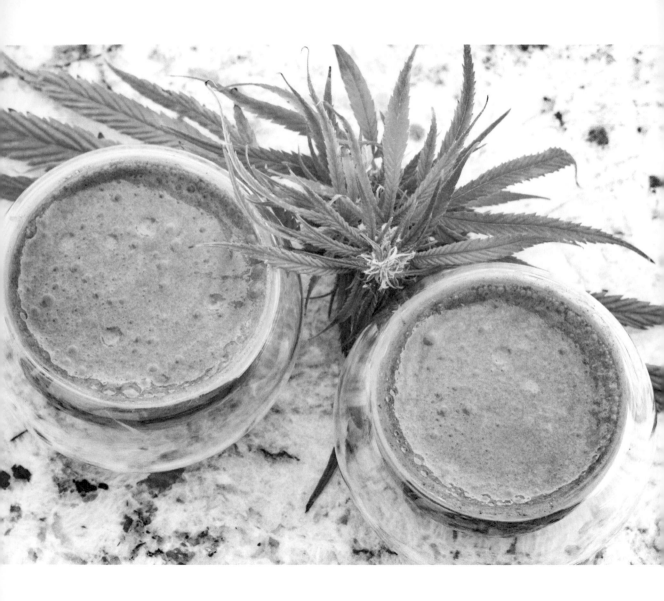

fully cover the plant material. Add enough cannabis and alcohol to fill the jar you have selected halfway. Do not fill more than halfway to give plenty of space inside to agitate the plant material. Use a second jar to make more, if necessary. Affix the lid tightly and give it a good shake.

3. Prepare a large pan with warm water. This water should be no warmer than 140° F (60° C). Place the jars with the alcohol and cannabis into the warm water and allow this to remain until the water cools to room temperature. Take the jar(s) out of the water and shake well.

4. Place the jar(s) on the counter, in a dark, warm spot, for at least a week. Shake once a day. I've left my tincture jars to infuse up to a month with terrific results.

5. Prepare a clean glass jar to decant your tincture. Use a funnel lined with cheesecloth to filter the plant material, if necessary. Filter the liquid tincture from the plant material into another clean jar or bowl.

6. Prepare your final tincture bottles. Using a funnel or other spout, fill each of the bottles and cap with the dropper caps. Use within 6 months for best results.

CBDA Tincturing

Tincturing CBDA does not require the decarboxylation process and retains more of the natural terpene content of the cannabis plant material you are using. This process works best when you can wait at least 2 weeks or more for your tincture to process.

Cured or fresh CBDA-rich cannabis flowers and leaves, or any sifted hashish
150-proof or higher culinary-grade alcohol
1 glass canning jar with sealable lid
Large pot to hold warm water
Funnel lined with cheesecloth
Glass tincture bottles with bulb dropper caps

1. Calculate the final concentration of CBDA, per serving, number of servings, and the serving size that you desire. The typical serving size of a dropperful is ¼ teaspoon to ⅔ teaspoon (1ml to 3ml). Since you will be working with high-proof alcohol, creating serving sizes that are no greater than 1 teaspoon (5ml), which is high in CBDA concentration,

is the best for ensuring alcohol consumption is negligible when using tinctures orally.

2. Select a glass canning jar that will be half full of cannabis and alcohol after everything has been added. Coarsely chop the cannabis material, and place it in the glass jar. Pour the alcohol over the cannabis material making sure that the cannabis material is completely covered. Affix the lid tightly and shake vigorously.

3. Prepare a large pan with warm water. The temperature of the water should be no higher than 140° F (60° C). Place the jars with the alcohol and cannabis into the warm water and allow this to remain until the water cools to room temperature. Take the jar(s) out of the water and shake well.

4. Place the jar(s) on the counter, in a dark, warm spot, for at least 2 weeks. Shake once a day.

5. Prepare a clean glass jar to decant your tincture. Use a funnel lined with cheesecloth to filter the plant material, if necessary. Filter the liquid tincture from the plant material into another clean jar or bowl.

6. Prepare your final tincture bottles. Using a funnel or other spout, fill each of the bottles and cap with the dropper caps. Use within 6 months for best results.

CBD Infusion for Beverage and Broth Recipe

Beverage infusion using tinctured CBD or CBDA and acacia gum powder is a convenient way to infuse CBD and CBDA into beverages—especially clear beverages and broth. High grades of acacia gum powder are best for all beverages, hot or cold. One serving of beverage or broth, for these purposes, is approximately 6 to 8 ounces (177ml–240ml).

CBD or CBDA tincture, 1 dropperful or up to 1 tsp (1ml–5ml), per beverage or broth serving

½ tsp–1 tsp (1g–2.5g) acacia gum powder, per beverage or broth serving

1 tbsp (15ml) room temperature water, per beverage or broth serving

1. Add the tincture and the acacia gum powder to each serving cup or bowl. Add the water.
2. Whisk vigorously until fully combined and emulsified.
3. Your serving cup or bowl is now ready for the beverage or broth you would like to add. Slowly add the beverage or broth while stirring. Serve immediately.

CBDA in The Raw Recipe

Juicing or otherwise incorporating fresh cannabis flowers and leaves is a fantastic method of enjoying everything the fresh cannabis plant has to offer. Fresh flowers and leaves are rich in CBDA, terpenes, fiber, vitamins, and minerals. You may obtain cuttings of mature plants or even grow a small cannabis plant that is rich in CBDA to the point that it develops a few flowers. To easily get the most of out your fresh plant material, you can juice or pulp it for smoothies now, or you can freeze it into cubes for use in juice or smoothies later.

Method 1:

Flowers and leaves can be directly juiced through a standard juicer if you have one. Juice and freeze the juice in an ice cube tray. Pop the juice out of the tray after it is frozen and store in a tightly closed freezer container.

Fresh CBD-rich cannabis flowers and leaves
A juicer or blender
Water
Ice cube tray
Freezer storage container

Method 2:

Use a blender and a little water to allow the material to fully pulp. Unlike juicing, this will retain all the fiber in the plant material. After blending into a smooth consistency, pour into ice cube trays and freeze immediately. After this has frozen solid, pop the cubes from the tray and store in a tightly closed freezer container.

Note:

A typical dose is 1 cube per juice or smoothie serving. More of the green flavor will come forward if you choose to use more cubes in your juices or smoothies.

CBD-like Alternative Herbs and Substitutions

In some locales, CBD is not available or, if it is, it is of very low quality. But did you know there are other plants with similar chemistry that are also helpful for relief and relaxation? Caryophyllene is a terpene that exists in cannabis flowers and has similar activity to cannabinoids like CBD and THC. Caryophyllene also exists in very rich amounts in cloves, black pepper, carnations, oregano, basil, hops, and many other plants that are easily accessible in locations where CBD may not be as accessible.

Research has shown that caryophyllene can bind to cannabinoid receptors.[11] Herbs, flowers, and foods with high amounts of this terpene are a good alternative to keep in mind when creating recipes with similar effectiveness to CBD.

Whenever possible, select the whole herb, spice, or flower to include in your recipes. Whole-plant aromatic infusion is discussed at length in the CBD Spa Time chapter that follows and is the best way to take advantage of this terpene and others found in whole aromatic plants.

Ingredient Sourcing

Many of the ingredients found in this book can be purchased at your local natural foods store. I have also included a Resources section after the last chapter of this book that includes all of my favorite online shops which carry many of the finest ingredients, such as Iranian saffron and rare varieties of frankincense resin, for example, that may be more difficult to source locally.

---

11 "Beta-caryophyllene is a dietary cannabinoid," *Proceedings of the National Academy of Sciences,* July 2008, Jürg Gertsch et al. 105 (26) 9099–9104; DOI: 10.1073/pnas.0803601105. https://www.ncbi.nlm.nih.gov/pmc/articles/PMC2449371/.

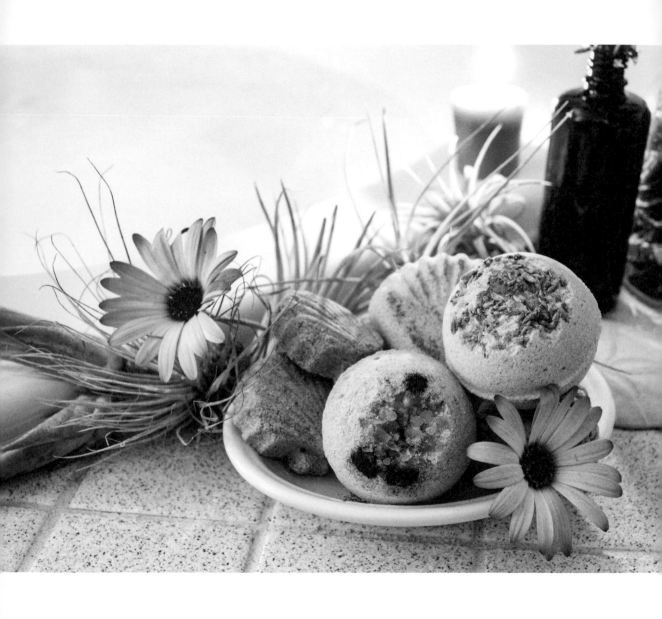

CHAPTER THREE

CBD SPA TIME

The Whole-Plant Aromatics Way

Essential oils have become a popular way to add fragrance and terpenes to spa preparations as makers have replaced artificial fragrances with these often costly, and very concentrated, forms of natural plant fragrance. In this chapter, in the spirit of the way of whole-plant extractions of CBD, whole-plant extractions of aromatic plants are favored over the use of essential oils.

The results are nothing short of spectacular. Whole aromatic plant infusion creates a much more expansive palette of fragrance experience—multidimensional, if you will. Fragrances are lighter and cleaner, but they are also more tenacious and vibrant than the distilled or solvent-extracted essential oils that you may be used to working with in your spa craft. The processes for creating these aromatic plant infusions are longer, but the results are worth the wait.

The fragrances I have experienced after moving away from essential oils and toward whole aromatic plant infusions in my cannabis spa craft have ethereal qualities not found in bottled essential oils; they capture the diversity of fragrance and the spirit of the plant as it exists in nature. I've noticed that my olfactory sensitivity for detecting subtlety has returned since working exclusively with whole-plant aromatics, and this is something I felt I was missing in my spa craft when I was using essential oils almost exclusively for fragrance and terpene infusion.

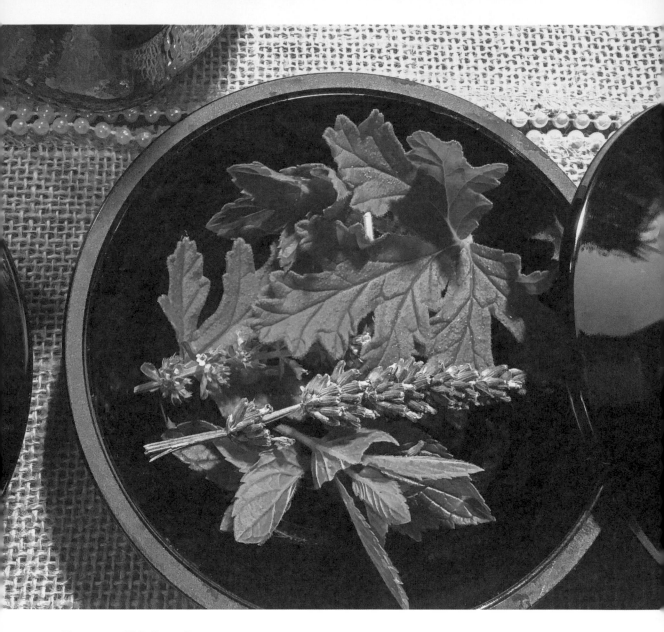

I am certain you will find deep satisfaction and a connection with the plants used to create the aroma experiences in this chapter. These complement whole-plant CBD infusions perfectly with an entourage of terpenes.

Working with Whole-Plant Aromatics

Whole-plant aromatics come in various forms: dried leafy, fruit, and flower plant material (dried mint, dried rosebuds, dried lavender flowers), dried barks or woody dried plant material (dried cinnamon sticks, cloves, peppercorns), resins and waxes (dried frankincense tears, myrrh resin, pine resin, bayberry wax, beeswax) and fresh forms, such as fresh aromatic leaves and flowers, fresh barks and needles, fresh citrus peel, and fresh resins scraped from trees and shrubs.

Any of these can be selected to create the blends of fragrance that you desire, keeping in mind that lotion and other skin preparations must be formulated as non-phototoxic. Certain plants can have a phototoxic effect; they create an extreme sensitivity to the sun. Typically, this is less of a problem with whole-plant aromatic infusions due to the much smaller amount of plant aromatics and a different combination of those constituents than in distilled or solvent-extracted essential oils. However, you will want to avoid or use minimal amounts of certain plants that are known to cause phototoxicity. Some of those include: almost all citrus, parsley, fennel, rue, cumin, angelica, and St. John's wort—but you should always research each ingredient you intend to add to your aromatic blend to ensure none are phototoxic and all are safe for use on the skin.

The Aromatic Formulation and Experience Vessel

Selection of the aromatic terpene blends that you prefer for your own CBD spa creations begins with a special tool and a method to create the fragrance and beneficial qualities that come with the entourage effect that you desire.

The key to creating the highest-quality whole-plant aromatic blends is the tool that you will use to create and sample these blends. My preference is the MIRON Violet Flame Glass charging bowl. These small bowls,

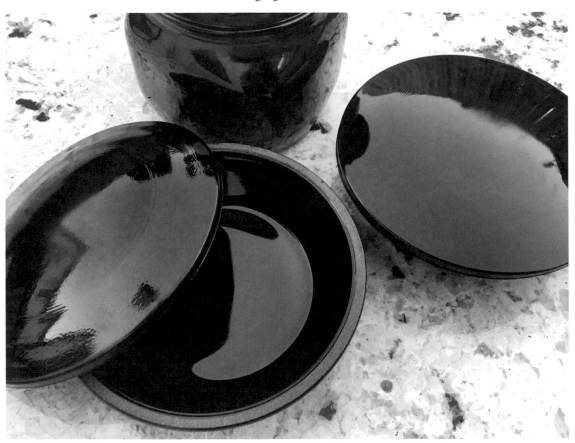

which hold approximately 300ml of liquid content, are composed of a kind of dark violet glass that allows for only the violet spectrum of light and infrared to penetrate through the glass. They are manufactured by only one scientific glass manufacturer—and are only available at select specialty stores as a retail product. The shape and functionality of these bowls make them the ideal tool to create and sample the aromatic whole-plant terpenes that you will be using in your own spa craft.

Alternatively, you can use amber glass canning jars to create and sample whole-plant aromatics. I prefer the MIRON glass charging bowls due to the shape of the bowl, which is ideal for capturing fragrance for sampling, as well as the functionality of the glass. But the amber glass canning jar would be my second choice—and these jars are available at most supermarkets. Avoid clear and other colored glass for best results.

To create and sample whole-plant aromatics, you will need:
1 or more MIRON Violet Flame Glass charging bowls with fitted glass lid, or an amber glass canning jar with a new lid
Fresh or dried herbs, resins, and waxes (Fresh herbs should be washed in cold, filtered water and completely dried.)
Scissors
Mortar and Pestle

1. Select the herbs that you would like to blend together. Select an amount of herbs that, when coarsely chopped and broken, will fill no more than half of the charging bowl or amber glass canning jar.
2. Weigh and measure each herb that you intend to add, separately, and write this number down.
3. Coarsely cut the fresh green herbs and flowers with scissors into the bowl or jar. Break up any large chunks of resin, wax, or bark into smaller pieces using a mortar and pestle or other hard surface suitable for this task, and add to the charging bowl or jar.
4. Add powdered herbs, small flowers, and herbs like lavender flowers or elderberry flowers last.
5. Gently combine, making sure the herbs are evenly distributed in the bowl or jar. Place the glass lid securely on the bowl or screw the lid firmly on to the jar.

You are now ready to use one or a combination of both methods to create your whole-plant aromatic blend:

1. Place the bowl or jar in a sunny location for 15 minutes to 1 hour. If you are in an especially hot climate or are using mostly fresh green herb and flower aromatics, 15 minutes should be enough time to fully mature the blend for sampling. Bark, resin, and some other dried or resinous aromatics may need more time to mature inside the charging bowl or jar. Generally speaking, if you are using an amber glass canning jar, it may need more time in the sun to mature the fragrance due to the size.

2. Place the bowl or jar on the counter in your kitchen or other warm room, and allow the fragrance to mature for 4 to 24 hours.

Sampling and editing the whole plant aromatic blend that you have created:

1. In an area free of other airborne fragrances, gently shake the bowl or jar and then partially slide the lid off your charging bowl, or partially remove the lid of the jar while bringing the fragrance up to your nose. Replace the lid on the bowl or jar. Wait at least 2 minutes.

2. Repeat a second time, sliding the lid off the bowl almost all the way, or removing the lid of the jar almost all the way while sampling the fragrance. Replace the lid on the bowl or jar.

3. If you like what you have created, note the amounts you wrote down earlier for each ingredient you have added to the charging bowl or jar. You will be adding these in the same proportions to the whole-plant aromatic infusion you want to create.

4. If you think something needs to be added, or increased, you can add to the bowl and follow the steps again from the beginning, gently combining the herbs and processing the fragrance to maturity in the covered charging bowl or jar.

5. If you feel that an ingredient needs to be omitted, you will need to wash your charging bowl or jar and begin again with fresh ingredients. If only some of an ingredient needs to be omitted, take out the amount

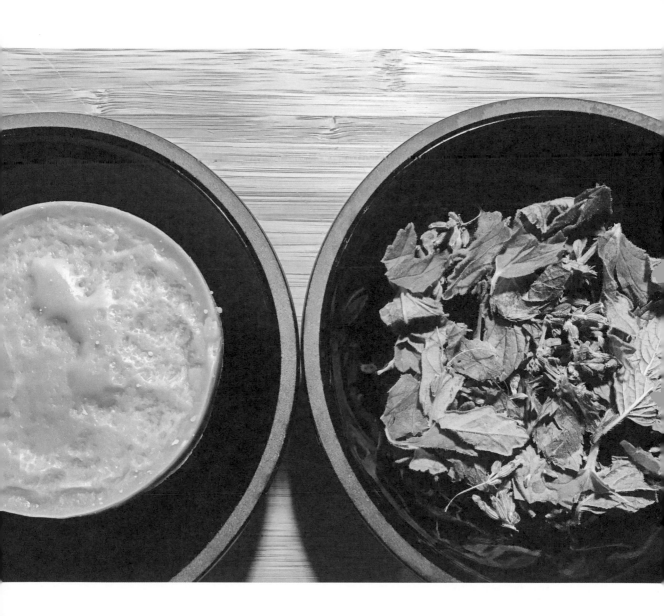

you want to omit, combine the ingredients again, gently and evenly distributing them, and replace the lid. Process again from step one.

*TIP The MIRON glass charging bowl is also a fantastic way to sample the fragrance notes and terpenes of any CBD-rich cannabis flower or sifted hashish. Place the cannabis plant material into the bowl and cover securely with the glass lid. Allow this to sit in a warm area such as the kitchen, covered, for 2 hours. Now you can sample the full range of terpene fragrances or pass the bowl around to guests to enjoy before vaporizing or smoking your CBD-rich flowers or hash.

Aromatics Infusion Methods

Aromatic plants can be infused for their fragrance and terpenes in a way similar to how we infuse cannabis for CBD and terpenes. Each of the CBD spa recipes in this book details the method for infusing the aromatic herbs that are called for in the individual recipe. Any of these recipes can have their aromatics replaced with the aromatic plants of your choosing! Select your favorite aromatics using the whole-plant aromatics formulation method described here.

Aromatic Oil Infusion

The aromatics that you infuse will serve as a base oil in your CBD spa recipes such as massage oil, salve, and lotion. There are two methods of whole-plant aromatic oil infusion that you will be working with in these recipes:

Water-Oil Infusion: For use with fresh, green plant material. **Excludes all resins, some barks, and saponin-producing herbs**.

Oil-Only Infusion: For use **only** with dried herbs, including resins, barks, and saponin-producing herbs.

To create a clean aromatic oil free of moisture, select the infusion method that is appropriate for the aromatic plant material you have on hand. If you have a mix of dried and fresh herbs, you will be using the water-oil infusion method. However, you would make sure to omit any aromatic herbs that have gums, saponins, or other chemistry that would emulsify the water and oil together. For example, you would not process frankincense or other tree resins using the water-oil infusion method due to emulsification of the gums, which would prevent the separation of the water from the oil at the end of the process.

Whole-Plant Aromatic Dry Salt and Soda Infusion

Some CBD spa recipes, such as bath salts or bath bombs, will call for infusing whole-plant aromatics into dry ingredients such as salt or sodium bicarbonate (soda). This can be achieved by processing dry aromatic plant ingredients, salt, or soda in heat or by grinding or otherwise combining the aromatic plants, whole, into the final product.

Aromatic Terpene Infusion of Cured CBD-rich Cannabis Flowers

Boosting the terpene content of your CBD-rich dried and cured cannabis flowers creates a delightful flavor and fragrance experience if you would like to also vaporize flower material during a spa session! Select any flavorful dried herb with the terpene content you desire, such as dried mint, lavender, orange peels, or pine needles. In an amber glass canning jar, generously pack these fragrant dried herbs around, bury your cannabis flowers in them, and fasten the lid tightly. It may be necessary to add a desiccant packet to absorb moisture in the jar if you are in a humid environment.

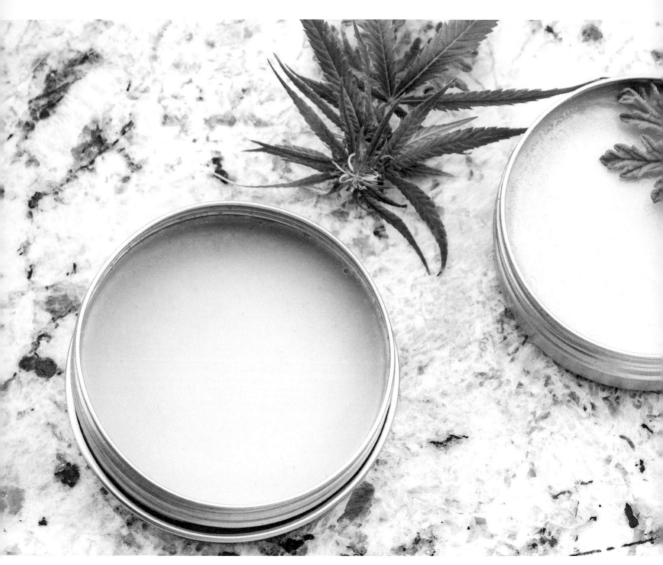

Farmer's Salve

Salves

Farmer's Salve

Geranium (*Pelargonium*) is a popular and easy-to-grow floral herb grown by many in the Emerald Triangle cannabis farming country of Northern California. *Pelargonium* is native to South Africa and has so many varieties! Scented Geranium a very diverse family within this species that has powerful fragrances ranging from rose, lemon, nutmeg, mint, pine, and more. Many of the same fragrant terpenes found in cannabis can also be found in the scented geranium. Geranium is also a much-loved herb for healing skin and topical preparations. Creating a fresh salve or lotion from this fragrant plant is always heavenly, and it will easily infuse into any oil you want to work with.

Makes 8 oz (240ml) of salve

1½ cups (100g) rose-scented geranium leaves and flowers, finely chopped, packed

½ cup (15g) fresh lemon thyme, finely chopped

½ cup (15g) fresh chamomile flowers, packed

½ cup (120ml) murumuru butter

¾ cup (180ml) distilled water

¼ cup (60ml) beeswax

⅓ cup (80ml) CBD-infused olive oil (see page 22 for making the CBD-infused olive oil

2g or 2ml of liquid sunflower lecithin

For the aromatic murumuru butter:

1. Fill a canning bath or stockpot with water. Prepare a clean glass canning jar and new lid. Wash all the herbs in cool water to remove debris and then chop the geranium and lemon thyme.

2. Add the distilled water and all herbs to the canning jar along with the murumuru butter. Affix the lid tightly and place in the canning bath or stockpot.

3. Bring the canning bath or stockpot to a simmer and process the jar for 30 minutes.

4. Turn off the heat and carefully remove the jar from the water. Allow it to cool until warm to the touch on a towel on the counter, but do not allow the oil to harden. Once the jar has cooled, carefully open it; it may have sealed during the processing of the oil.

5. Strain the water and oil from the herbs through cheesecloth and gently squeeze to release as much of the oil and water from the plant material

as possible into a glass jar or bowl. Allow this to sit on the counter for 10 minutes while the oil and water separate.

6. Place the jar or bowl, covered, in the freezer for about 10 minutes just to harden the murumuru butter on top of the liquid before it begins to freeze. Remove this from the freezer and cut the hardened oil from the top of the jar or bowl, leaving the water behind. Discard the water. Place the hardened disk of oil you have just removed from the jar or bowl with the side that had been touching the water down on a clean towel to quickly absorb all the moisture left on the bottom of the oil. Use the towel to remove all debris and moisture.

7. The hardened and dried murumuru butter is now fully infused with the fragrances and properties of the fresh herbs and is ready to use in this salve.

Make the salve:

1. In a pan on low heat, melt the beeswax with the CBD-infused olive oil and sunflower lecithin. Add the aromatic murumuru butter and remove from the heat as soon as it has melted completely into the wax and CBD-infused olive oil. Stir.

2. Pour the mixture immediately into a clean glass or metal salve container. Rest on the counter for 5 minutes, affix the lid, and then place in the freezer for 15 to 20 minutes to fully harden. The freezer step is necessary to prevent the salve having a grainy texture.

3. Remove from the freezer and the salve is ready to use and shelf-stable. Use within 6 months for best results.

Wild Emerald Herbs Salve

Inspired by the mountains and forests of the Emerald Triangle cannabis-growing regions of California, balsam, pine, and the skin-soothing properties of blackberry leaf come together with whole-plant CBD infusion in MCT oil. This recipe uses the special, long-process CBD Farmer's Oil Recipe with Whole Flowers from page 18. This recipe, like many others in this chapter, uses pure bayberry wax, an aromatic vegan wax obtained by boiling the berries of the Myrica tree.

Makes: 8 oz (240ml) of salve

½ cup (15g) dried blackberry leaves, crushed

1 cup (40g) dried pine needles and resin, crushed and broken

½ cup (120ml) murumuru butter

¼ cup (60ml) bayberry wax

¼ cup (60ml) CBD-infused MCT oil (see page 18 for making the CBD Farmer's Oil Recipe with Whole Flowers)

2g or 2ml liquid sunflower lecithin

For the aromatic murumuru butter:

1. Fill a canning bath or stockpot with water. Prepare a clean glass canning jar and new lid. Crush the blackberry leaves, pine needles, and pine resin using a mortar and pestle.
2. Add all herbs to the canning jar along with the murumuru butter. Affix the lid tightly and place in the canning bath or stockpot.
3. Bring the canning bath or stockpot to a simmer and process the jar for 30 minutes.
4. Turn off the heat and carefully remove the jar from the water. Allow it to cool until warm to the touch on a towel on the counter, but do not allow the oil to harden. Once the jar has cooled sufficiently, carefully open it; it may have sealed during the processing of the oil.
5. Strain the oil from the herbs through cheesecloth and gently squeeze to release as much of the oil from the plant material as possible into a glass jar or bowl.
6. The aromatic herb-infused murumuru butter is ready to use in this salve.

Make the salve:

1. In a pan on low heat, melt the bayberry wax with the CBD-infused MCT oil and sunflower lecithin. Add the aromatic murumuru butter

and remove from the heat as soon as it has melted completely into the wax and CBD-infused MCT oil. Stir.

2. Pour the mixture immediately into a clean glass or metal salve container. Rest on the counter for 5 minutes, affix the lid, and then place in the freezer for 15 to 20 minutes to fully harden. The freezer step is necessary to prevent the salve having a grainy texture.

3. Remove from the freezer and the salve is ready to use and shelf-stable. Use within 6 months for best results.

Minty Chocolate Lip Balm

Making lip balm is a totally delicious way to use your CBD-infused coconut oil! This recipe infuses mint flavor directly into cacao butter for a fragrant and tasty chocolate mint flavor every time you use this on your lips. Apply as often as you like for flavor, moisture, and the benefits of CBD. Makes a great lip balm for the winter season.

Makes 4oz (120ml) of lip balm

½ cup (15g) mint leaves, or chocolate mint–scented geranium leaves, dried and crushed

5 tbsp + 1 tsp (70ml) cacao butter

3 tbsp + 1 tsp (50ml) CBD-infused coconut oil (page 25)

1g or 1ml liquid sunflower lecithin

For the mint cacao butter:

1. Fill a canning bath or stockpot with water. Prepare a clean glass canning jar and new lid. Crush the dried mint or mint-scented geranium leaves using a mortar and pestle.
2. Add the crushed leaves to the canning jar along with the cacao butter. Affix the lid tightly and place in the canning bath or stockpot.
3. Bring the canning bath or stockpot to a simmer and process the jar for 30 minutes.
4. Turn off the heat and carefully remove the jar from the water. Allow it to cool until warm to the touch on a towel on the counter, but do not allow the oil to harden. Once the jar has cooled sufficiently, carefully open it; it may have sealed during the processing of the oil.
5. Strain the oil from the leaves through cheesecloth and gently squeeze to release as much of the oil from the plant material as possible into a small pan.

Make the lip balm:

1. Prepare the lip balm containers that you would like to use.
2. Add the CBD-infused coconut oil and sunflower lecithin to the pan with the mint-infused cacao butter. Warm to melt everything together and stir to combine.

3. Pour the lip balm into the lip balm containers. Allow to cool for 5 minutes on the counter and then transfer to the freezer to cool the lip balm until hardened, about 20 minutes. The balm will be shelf-stable and solid at room temperature afterward. The freezer step is necessary to prevent a grainy texture in the finished lip balm. Use within 6 months for best results.

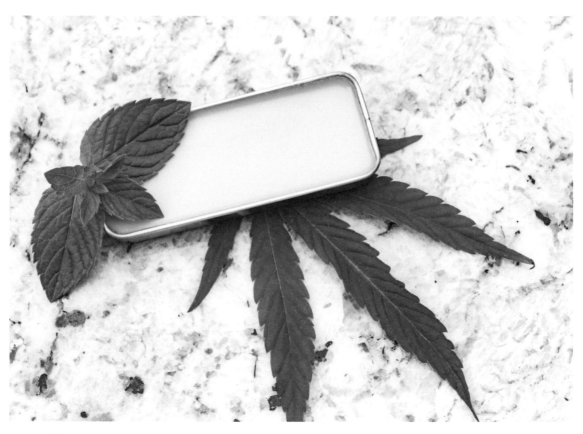

Minty Chocolate Lip Balm

Whipped Chocolate Body Butter

A delicious body butter that feels as great as it smells and tastes! Yes, you can taste this one! There's more than one way to make this body butter, so if you'd like something a bit more warming and pain-relieving, as well as fragrant, try making this with cinnamon and hot pepper! You will need a hand mixer or a stand mixer to get the "whipped" texture you desire. This butter should be kept in a cool environment so that it maintains the light whipped texture.

Makes: 8oz (240ml) body butter

1 whole vanilla bean, chopped
1 tsp (3g) whole cacao nibs
⅓ cup (80ml) cacao butter
⅓ cup (80ml) sunflower oil
⅓ cup (80ml) CBD-infused coconut oil (page 25)
2g or 2ml liquid sunflower lecithin
Optional for a warming and pain-relieving chocolate body butter:
1 or more cinnamon sticks or pieces
1 or more whole dried hot pepper

For the aromatic chocolate butter:

1. Fill a canning bath or stockpot with water. Prepare a clean glass canning jar and new lid. Prepare the chopped vanilla bean and cacao nibs along with cinnamon sticks and hot peppers if you would like to add those, as well. Remember when working with hot peppers to wash your hands before touching your eyes or other mucous membranes.
2. Add the herbs to the canning jar along with the cacao butter, and sunflower oil. Affix the lid tightly and place in the canning bath or stockpot.
3. Bring the canning bath or stockpot to a simmer and process the jar for 30 minutes.
4. Turn off the heat and carefully remove the jar from the water. Allow it to cool until warm to the touch on a towel on the counter, but do not allow the oil to harden. Once the jar has cooled sufficiently, carefully open it; it may have sealed during the processing of the oil.
5. Strain the oil from the leaves through cheesecloth and gently squeeze to release as much of the oil from the plant material as possible into a small pan.

Make the body butter:

1. Add the CBD-infused coconut oil and sunflower lecithin to the pan with the oil that has been strained. Gently melt everything together and combine thoroughly.

2. Using stainless-steel pans for the whipping process will give the best results, as they retain and hold the cold temperature needed to whip the oils into a body butter. You can begin to cool the pan in the refrigerator until the contents are not quite solid but can still be whipped with a mixer. Or you can double the pan by placing it in another pan filled with ice and whipping it while it sits atop the ice.

3. Once the mixture has been prepared for whipping by using one of the methods in step 2, whip the butter using a mixer until it is fluffy, light, and fairly solid. It should have stiff peaks and remain light and fluffy.

4. Scoop the finished butter into the jar you have prepared for your body butter. Place this into the refrigerator for 5 to 10 minutes to fully set. Afterward, it will be shelf-stable if kept in a cool environment. Should your butter melt at any time, you can re-whip into light fluffy butter again by following the steps in this recipe. Use within 3 months for best results.

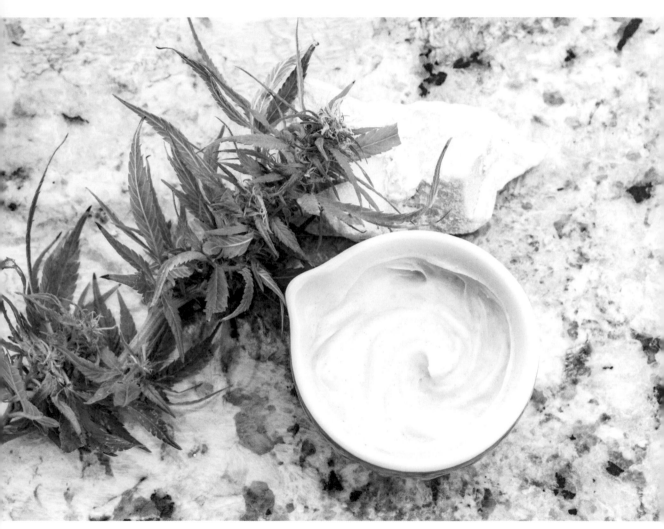

Whipped Chocolate Body Butter

Oklahoma Rose Beauty Cream

This is quite possibly the most exquisite whipped beauty cream I have ever made—and I think you will agree that it is indeed a special spa treat unlike anything else you've ever tried! Inspired by the Oklahoma rose (the official flower of the state of Oklahoma), I formulated this recipe while growing this deep red rose with an extraordinary rose fragrance in my own garden. When I first encountered this rose, I knew it had exactly the qualities I wanted for a beauty cream. Not everyone will have this rose in their garden, but you can use any highly fragrant fresh pink or red rose to make this beauty cream.

Makes: 8oz (240ml) beauty cream

For the rose-infused aromatic murumuru butter:

1. Fill a canning bath or stockpot with water. Prepare a clean glass canning jar and new lid. Wash the roses in cool water, remove all the petals, and discard the cores. This recipe uses petals only.
2. Add the culinary rose water and the rose petals to the canning jar along with the murumuru butter. Affix the lid tightly and place in the canning bath or stock pan.
3. Bring the canning bath or stockpot to a simmer and process the jar for 30 minutes.
4. Turn off the heat and carefully remove the jar from the water. Allow it to cool until warm to the touch on a towel on the counter, but do not allow the oil to harden. Once the jar has cooled, carefully open it; it may have sealed during the processing of the oil.
5. Strain the water and oil from the herbs through cheesecloth and gently squeeze to release as much of the oil and water from the rose petals as possible into a glass jar or bowl. Allow this to sit on the counter for 10 minutes while the oil and water separate.

12 or more large, fresh Oklahoma roses or another very fragrant rose, organic

⅓ cup (80ml) distilled culinary rose water

½ cup (120ml) murumuru butter

½ cup (120ml) CBD-infused camellia seed oil (page 22)

3 tbsp (45ml) bayberry wax

2g or 2ml liquid sunflower lecithin

6. Place the jar or bowl, covered, in the freezer for about 10 minutes just to harden the murumuru butter on top of the liquid before it begins to freeze. Remove this from the freezer and cut the hardened oil from the top of the jar or bowl, leaving the water behind. Discard the water. Place the hardened disk of oil you have just removed from the jar or bowl with the side that had been touching the water down on a clean towel to quickly absorb all the moisture left on the bottom of the oil. Use the towel to remove all debris and moisture.

Make the beauty cream:
1. Add the CBD-infused camellia seed oil, bayberry wax, and sunflower lecithin to a pan. Warm gently to combine thoroughly. Melt the rose-infused murumuru butter into this mixture and remove from the heat source as soon as everything is melted together.
2. Using stainless-steel pans for the whipping process will give the best results, as they retain and hold the cold temperature needed to whip this into a fluffy beauty cream. You can begin to cool the pan in the refrigerator until it is not quite solid but can still be whipped with a mixer. Or, you can double the pan by placing it in another pan filled with ice and whipping it while it sits in the pan with ice.
3. Once the mixture is ready to whip by using one of the methods in step 2, whip the beauty cream using a mixer until it is fluffy, light, and creamy.
4. Scoop the finished beauty cream into the jar you have prepared. Place this into the refrigerator for 5 to 10 minutes to fully set. Afterward, it will be shelf-stable if kept in a cool environment. Use within 3 months for best results.

Skin-Renewing Rose Hip Scrub

This is a totally refreshing salt scrub recipe that is somewhere between a moisturizing oil scrub and a clay mask. This special scrub exfoliates your skin with the power of rose hips, clay, and salt, while moisturizing and soothing with CBD-infused olive oil. Use before a shower or bath for the best results.

Makes: 8oz (240ml) scrub

1. Prepare a clean glass jar to store your scrub and set aside. In a small bowl, combine the powdered clay and rose hip powder. Pour the CBD-infused olive oil over this and work the oil into the powder thoroughly.
2. Add the salt to this mixture and work into the powder and oil. Once everything is combined evenly, scoop the mixture into the jar for final storage. Use within 3 months for best results.
3. To use this scrub, put some in a small bowl and mix with a little bit of culinary floral water until it becomes a paste. Spread over your skin and massage it in a circular motion. You may leave it on your skin for a few minutes before you shower or bathe.
4. Do not mix the floral water with the scrub until you actually use the scrub. The scrub is shelf-stable only until water is added.

½ cup (65g) Moroccan rhassoul clay powder

¼ cup (20g) rose hip powder

¼ cup (120ml) CBD-infused olive oil (page 22)

⅓ cup (80g) fine-grain sea salt

Culinary orange flower water or rose water

Balms

Super Pain Balm

A spicy and warm pain balm that is two recipes in one! This solid balm is portable and great to have for aches and pains from physical activity such as sports, hikes, or farming. It provides fast relief for joint and muscle pain of any kind. I'm quite fond of both of these herbal blends, as I've used both with similar soothing results.

Makes: 8oz (240ml) solid balm

For the spiced aromatic coconut oil:

1 handful (about 50g) of whole dried spice blends: cloves, black peppercorn, ginger OR turmeric, boswellia serrata, black peppercorn (This will lend a slight golden color to the skin when applied.) Blend the spices as you desire with the fragrance profile that you prefer using the aromatic discovery techniques described earlier in this chapter.
⅓ cup (80ml) coconut oil
3 tbsp (45ml) beeswax
½ cup (120ml) CBD-infused murumuru butter (page 25)
2g or 2ml liquid sunflower lecithin

1. Fill a canning bath or stockpot with water. Prepare a clean glass canning jar and new lid. Add the whole dried spices of your choice to the canning jar along with the coconut oil. Affix the lid tightly and place in the canning bath or stockpot.
2. Bring the canning bath or stockpot to a simmer and process the jar for 45 minutes.
3. Turn off the heat and carefully remove the jar from the water. Allow it to cool until warm to the touch on a towel on the counter, but do not allow the oil to harden. Once the jar has cooled sufficiently, carefully open it; it may have sealed during the processing of the oil.
4. Strain the oil from the herbs through cheesecloth and gently squeeze to release as much of the oil from the spices as possible into the small pan that you will use to make the balm.

Make the balm:

1. In the pan with the spiced coconut oil, apply low heat and melt the beeswax, CBD-infused murumuru butter, and the sunflower lecithin together with the spiced coconut oil, combining thoroughly.

2. Pour the mixture immediately into balm containers. Rest on the counter for 5 minutes, affix the lid, and then place in the freezer for 20 minutes to fully harden. The freezer step is necessary to prevent the balm having a grainy texture.
3. Remove from the freezer and the balm is ready to use and is shelf-stable. Use within 6 months for best results.

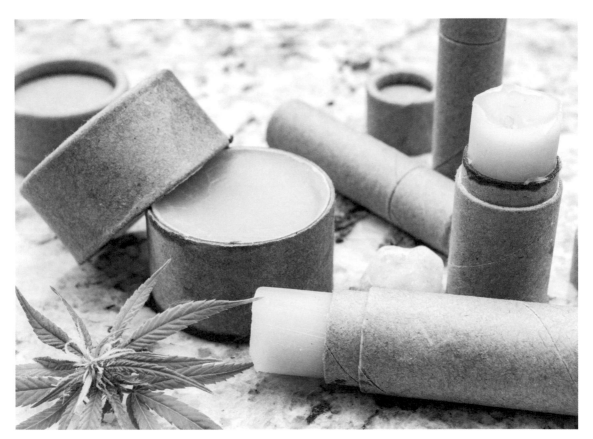

Super Pain Balm

Ave Maria Balm

I was inspired to make this balm one afternoon while working in my kitchen and listening to the classical violin composition of "Ave Maria." Its balsamic, resinous, and old-fashioned floral aromas remind me of old churches and holy places. It's a nice balm for applying to temples and other pressure points for its meditative and relaxing effects.

Makes: 8oz (240ml) solid balm

For the aromatic murumuru butter:

2 tbsp (20g) frankincense frereana resin
2 tsp (7g) myrrh resin
1 tbsp (12g) benzoin styrax resin
¼ cup (20g) dried Turkish rosebuds and petals
½ cup (120ml) murumuru butter
¼ cup (60ml) bayberry wax
¼ cup (60ml) CBD-infused olive oil (page 22)
2g or 2ml liquid sunflower lecithin

1. Fill a canning bath or stockpot with water. Prepare a clean glass canning jar and new lid. Add the resins and rosebuds to the jar along with the murumuru butter and affix the lid tightly. Place the jar into the canning bath or stockpot.
2. Bring the canning bath or stockpot to a simmer and process the jar for 45 minutes.
3. Turn off the heat and carefully remove the jar from the water. Allow it to cool until warm to the touch on a towel on the counter, but do not allow the oil to harden. Once the jar has cooled sufficiently, carefully open it; it may have sealed during the processing of the oil.
4. Strain the oil from the herbs through cheesecloth and gently squeeze to release as much of the oil from the herbs as possible into the small pan that you will use to make the balm.

Continued on page 64.

Make the balm:

1. In the pan with the aromatic murumuru, apply low heat and melt the bayberry wax, CBD-infused olive oil, and the sunflower lecithin together with the aromatic murumuru butter, combining thoroughly.
2. Pour the mixture immediately into balm containers. Rest on the counter for 5 minutes, affix the lid, and then place in the freezer for 20 minutes to fully harden. The freezer step is necessary to prevent the balm having a grainy texture.
3. Remove from the freezer and the balm is ready to use and is shelf-stable. Use within 6 months for best results.

Massage Oil and Honey

Sun Salute Massage Oil

This recipe features a rare form of frankincense called blue/green frankincense sacra. I discovered it on one of my spa-crafting adventures. This resin is difficult to find, but well worth it, as it is a rare collection of frankincense resin obtained from the top of the tree. Combined with lavender flowers or mint leaves and CBD-infused camellia seed oil, this massage oil is refreshing and invigorating—perfect for yoga and any morning stretching routine.

Makes: 8oz (240ml) massage oil

For the aromatic rice bran oil:

2 tbsp (20g) frankincense sacra (rare blue/green variety if you can find it!)

¼ cup (15g) dried lavender flowers or mint leaves

½ cup (120ml) rice bran oil

⅓ cup (80ml) CBD-infused camellia seed oil (page 22)

3 tbsp (45ml) bayberry wax

2g or 2ml liquid sunflower lecithin

1. Fill a canning bath or stockpot with water. Prepare a clean glass canning jar and new lid. Add the herbs to the jar along with the rice bran oil and affix the lid tightly. Place the jar into the canning bath or stockpot.
2. Bring the canning bath or stockpot to a simmer and process the jar for 45 minutes.
3. Turn off the heat and carefully remove the jar from the water. Allow it to cool until warm to the touch on a towel on the counter. Once the jar has cooled sufficiently, carefully open it; it may have sealed during the processing of the oil.
4. Strain the oil from the herbs through cheesecloth and gently squeeze to release as much of the oil from the herbs as possible into the small pan that you will use to make the massage oil.

Make the massage oil:

1. In the pan with the aromatic rice bran oil, apply low heat, and melt the CBD-infused camellia seed oil, bayberry wax, and the

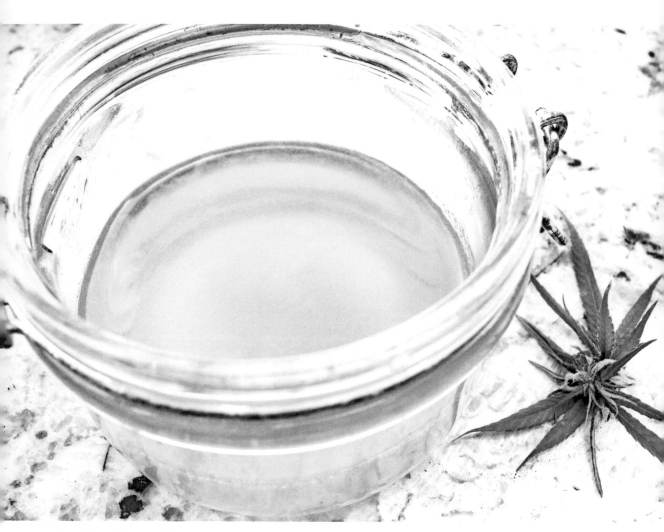

Sun Salute Massage Oil

sunflower lecithin together with the aromatic rice bran oil, combining thoroughly.

2. Pour the mixture immediately into a clean glass bottle, and affix the lid or pump to the bottle. Rest on the counter for 5 minutes, shake the contents, and then transfer to the refrigerator for 10 minutes or until the massage oil cools completely and becomes a little thicker.

3. Remove from the refrigerator. Shake the bottle again. Use within 3 months for best results.

Deep Relief Massage Honey

This massage "honey" is so rich and decadent, you'll think it looks just like honey when you pour it into the palm of your hand! It's made with beeswax, which gives it a honey-like aroma, along with the other sweet herbs, which are blended with CBD-infused oil that has been made with sifted hash. Your final massage honey will be the color of honey and just as sweet!

Makes: 8oz (240ml) massage "honey"

For the aromatic camellia seed oil:

1. Fill a canning bath or stockpot with water. Prepare a clean glass canning jar and new lid. Add the herbs to the jar along with the camellia seed oil and affix the lid tightly. Place the jar into the canning bath or stockpot.
2. Bring the canning bath or stockpot to a simmer and process the jar for 45 minutes.
3. Turn off the heat and carefully remove the jar from the water. Allow it to cool until warm to the touch on a towel on the counter. Once the jar has cooled sufficiently, carefully open it; it may have sealed during the processing of the oil.
4. Strain the oil from the herbs through cheesecloth and gently squeeze to release as much of the oil from the herbs as possible into the small pan that you will use to make the massage honey.

Make the massage honey:

1. In the pan with the aromatic camellia seed oil, apply low heat, and melt the CBD-infused murumuru butter, beeswax, and the sunflower lecithin together with the aromatic camellia seed oil, combining thoroughly.

3 tbsp (35g) frankincense serrata
½ vanilla bean, chopped
10 threads high-grade saffron
¼ cup (15g) dried scented geranium leaves (fruit or rose). Substitution with dried orange peels is also nice, but limit sun exposure after using this massage oil if you use citrus.
¾ cup (180ml) camellia seed oil (page 22)
3 tbsp (45ml) CBD-infused murumuru butter (made with sifted hash for best results in this recipe, page 25)
1 tbsp (15ml) beeswax
2g or 2ml liquid sunflower lecithin

2. Pour the mixture immediately into a clean glass bottle, and affix the lid or pump to the bottle. Rest on the counter for 5 minutes, shake the contents, and then transfer to the refrigerator for 10 minutes or until the massage honey thickens. Shake the bottle again.
3. Remove from the refrigerator. Refrigeration is suggested to create a smooth, lotion-like massage honey, but the final massage honey is shelf-stable once it has been processed. Use within 3 months for best results.

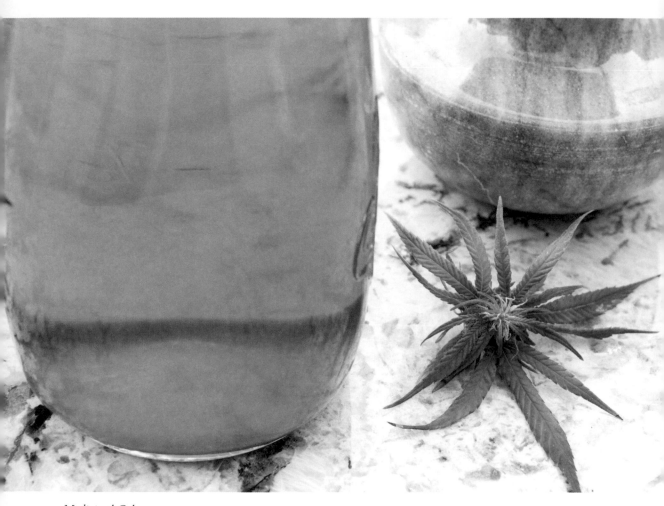

Medicinal Cologne

The Medicinal Cologne

Medicinal colognes have been around since at least the seventeenth century and are recorded in many herbal and medical texts. One of the more popular ones of the eighteenth century, 4711, was developed in Cologne, Germany, by Wilhelm Muelhens. This cologne is still sold today, albeit a somewhat different composition than the original recipe, as many colognes were intended in that time period for both external and internal use.

This CBDA-infused, whole-plant medicinal cologne is true to its roots; colognes developed hundreds of years ago were meant to refresh, soothe, and relieve both internally and externally. Part medicinal tincture, part aromatherapeutics—see if you don't fall in love with these as an everyday remedy.

These are rich in alcohol—no more than 2 ml is suggested for internal use. May be used generously as a body splash or on a cool wet cloth for relief from heat. They are great to add to water for a quick cleanup of face, neck, hands, and arms after outdoor activities too. I personally love to splash this cologne for immediate relief of hot flashes!

Plants with cooling properties are suggested for this recipe. Cool frankincense resin like frankincense sacra, scented geranium leaves, white tea, mint, rose petals, lavender flowers, lemon thyme, lemon balm, and basil, are among my favorites and are all edible. If you opt to use citrus peels or other potentially phototoxic herbs, avoid the sun after using this cologne externally.

Makes: 12oz (360ml) cologne

1 handful (100g) or a little more fresh or dried fragrant herbs and flowers.

5g–10g dried and cured CBDA-rich cannabis flowers (not decarboxylated)

1¼ cup (300ml) 150-proof or higher culinary-grade alcohol

¼ cup (60ml) distilled water (I like to use distilled culinary rose or orange flower water, but plain distilled water is fine)

1. In a large amber glass canning jar with a new lid, pack the herbs and CBD-rich cannabis flowers tightly. Leave at least 3 inches (7.5cm) at the top of the jar, but don't leave too much more than that—you will want to pack a generous amount of herbs into the jar for very fragrant cologne!

2. Pour the alcohol over the herbs until it is approximately 1 inch (2.5cm) above the herbs in the jar. With all of the herbs and alcohol in the jar, there should now be about a 2-inch (5cm) space left at the top of the jar.
3. Affix the lid tightly. Allow the jar to sit in a dark but warm area like the corner of the kitchen. Shake the jar at least 2 times a week for about 3 weeks. You can mature the jar even up to 6 weeks before you decant it.
4. Strain the liquid through a cheesecloth into a glass bowl, squeezing out as much liquid from the herbs as you can. Add the plain distilled water, or culinary rose or orange flower water for even more fragrance, and stir.
5. Prepare the final glass bottle that you will store your cologne in. Using a funnel, pour the liquid into the bottle and cap. Use within 6 months for best results.

Aromatic Herbal Soap

Handmade CBD-infused herbal soap isn't as hard as it sounds and uses very simple ingredients. This soap follows a similar aromatic plant infusion process as the salve and cream recipes in this chapter. Quick processing is done using the hot-process method, which takes about a week to cure, instead of a cold processing, which takes three to six months to cure. You can cold-process this soap by skipping the cooking process here and pouring directly into molds. Another advantage of cooking the soap is that it can be fashioned into soap spheres or other shapes after the cooking process but before it becomes completely hard.

You will need protective gloves, eyewear, and a face mask to work with lye. Outside is the ideal place to mix lye (a caustic chemical) before it is added to the oils.

Makes: 4–8 soap bars or spheres, depending on size

Assorted dried aromatic herbs and resins of your choice. Approximately 1 cup or more (60g–150g). Use the aromatic discovery method described in this chapter to select your aromatic palette for this soap.

8 oz (240ml) olive oil

2 oz (60ml) CBD-infused olive oil (page 22)

1 oz (30ml) hemp seed oil

5 oz (150ml) coconut oil

6.08 oz (180ml) cold distilled water, plain or distilled culinary rose or orange flower water that has no citric acid or other additives in the water

65g pure soapmakers' lye

For the aromatic olive oil:

1. Fill a canning bath or stockpot with water. Prepare a clean glass canning jar and new lid. Add the aromatic herbs and resins to the jar along with the olive oil and affix the lid tightly. Place the jar into the canning bath or stockpot.

2. Bring the canning bath or stockpot to a simmer and process the jar for 30 to 45 minutes.

3. Turn off the heat and carefully remove the jar from the water. Allow it to cool until warm to the touch on a towel on the counter. Once the jar has cooled sufficiently, carefully open it; it may have sealed during the processing of the oil.

4. Strain the oil from the herbs through cheesecloth and gently squeeze to release as much of the oil from the herbs as possible into a clean bowl.

Make the soap:

1. In a glass or ceramic container (do not use metal containers or implements), pour the cold distilled water, the distilled culinary rose water, or the orange flower water (whichever you desire). Put on your gloves and eyewear. Using a gram scale, measure the exact amount of lye called for in this recipe.

2. Slowly add the lye to the cold water while stirring. The water will heat up during this process—do not be alarmed. Continue to stir until all the lye crystals are dissolved completely. There should be no floating white specks or other sediment in the container. When the lye is fully dissolved, the water will begin to cool a bit. At this point, it is ready to add to the oils to make the soap. This process typically takes 15 minutes or a little longer.

3. In a slow cooker set on low, add the aromatic olive oil, the CBD-infused olive oil, the hemp seed oil, and the coconut oil. Stir and melt everything together to combine thoroughly. Once this has melted together, turn off the slow cooker; it is ready for the lye.

4. Slowly add the lye to the oils while stirring. Using a stick blender, begin to mix the oil and lye together until it reaches a trace. Trace will be when the oil and lye fully combine and resemble pancake batter.

5. Once the mixture has reached trace, you can pour into molds for cold processing of the soap bars. The soap bars should set up within 1 to 3 days and should be popped from the mold at that time, wrapped loosely in cheesecloth, and cured in a spot with good air circulation. The curing process will take 3 to 6 months. The longer cold-processed soap is cured, the higher quality it will be.

6. To hot process, continue stirring or using the stick blender and turn up your slow cooker to high for 15 minutes, and then back to low for the remaining 20 to 30 minutes it will take to process the soap. The soap is completed when it becomes the consistency of mashed potatoes. Some

soap makers will taste a bit on their tongue for the tell-tale *zap* that indicates that the soap is not quite ready. Generally speaking, the consistency of mashed potatoes will indicate a complete soap that can then be molded or shaped into spheres and then cured for 1 week before it is ready to use. Always wear gloves while handling soap before it is completely cured.

7. When the soap has finished curing, wrap in paper or cloth and keep in a cool and dry area. Most soap, cold or hot process, has a good shelf life of a year or a little longer.

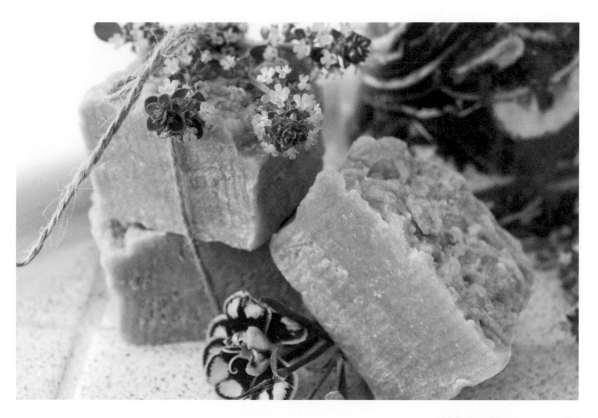

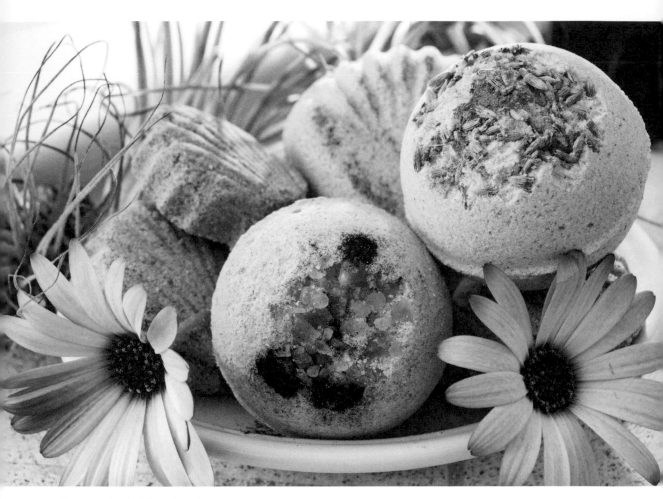

Fragrant Herbal Bath Bombs

2 cups (460g) sodium bicarbonate (culinary baking soda)

1 cup (211g) fine-grain Himalayan salt

½ cup (57g) soapwort root (Saponaria *officinalis*), powdered (no substitutions)

Whole, unbroken, dried aromatic resins and herbs to create the fragrance profile you desire.

1 tbsp (15 ml) or less CBD-infused high oleic acid oil such as camellia, olive, or rice bran (page 22) (a concentrated, sifted hash-infused oil is suggested for best results with this recipe)

1 cup (195g) citric acid

1 tbsp (8g) aloe vera, powdered

1 tsp (4g) benzoin styrax, powdered

Optional: Any powdered aromatic herbs, no more than 1 tbsp (10g)

80-proof or more culinary alcohol or the Medicinal Cologne recipe (pg 71), in a spray bottle

Bath bomb molds

Parchment paper and a drying tray

Fragrant Herbal Bath Bombs

I'm not one to brag, but I think this is going to become your favorite bath bomb recipe! It's been a favorite at the farmers' markets where I've had the privilege of sharing the non-cannabis formulation. It's specifically made to accommodate full emulsification and distribution of oils and resins throughout the water for a truly therapeutic, CBD-infused bathing experience.

Make sure the salt you use is "dry" and does not have significant amounts of magnesium, as are found in Epsom salt or Dead Sea salt, as this can attract additional moisture and activate bath bombs in the presence of humidity.

Makes about 3–10 bath bombs or tablets, depending on size

Make the infused aromatics salt mixture:

1. Fill a canning bath or stockpot with water. Prepare a clean glass canning jar and new lid. Make sure this is very dry before starting.

2. In a glass or ceramic bowl, mix the sodium bicarbonate, salt, and soapwort root together until thoroughly combined. Begin layering the whole aromatic herbs and resins and the salt mixture in the jar by starting with a layer of aromatics and then a layer of the salt mixture in roughly even amounts until the jar is completely layered with only 1 inch (2.5cm) left at the top. Affix the lid tightly. Do not shake. Place the jar into the canning bath or stockpot.

3. Bring the canning bath or stockpot to a simmer and process the jar for 45 minutes.

4. Turn off the heat and carefully remove the jar from the water. Allow it to cool completely on a towel on the counter. Once the jar has cooled completely, carefully open it; it may have sealed during the processing of the salt mixture.

5. Separate the plant material and salt mixture into two bowls made of glass or ceramic. Spoon each layer out into its respective bowl. The

plant material bowl may have some of the salt mixture; sift this out using a strainer into the salt mixture bowl. It is okay if there are pieces of plant material left in your salt mixture. Your aromatic salt mixture is now ready to make into bath bombs. The leftover plant material can be crushed or otherwise turned into decorative aromatic toppings for your bath bombs as seen in the photos here.

Make the bath bombs:

1. In the bowl with the aromatic salt mixture you have just processed, add the CBD-infused oil that you have selected and work this into the salt mixture to distribute it evenly.

2. Add the citric acid, powdered aloe vera, powdered benzoin styrax, and any powdered aromatic herbs you would like to add to the bath bombs and thoroughly combine with the salt mixture.

3. Using the alcohol or cologne in the spray bottle, spritz the mixture a couple times and then use your gloved hands to combine this with the dry mixture. The mixture should be spritzed just enough to make it slightly moist like sand and stick together when pressed in your hand.

4. In the bath bomb molds, add a little bit of the crushed herbs from making your aromatic salt to decorate the outside of your bath bombs if you desire. Fill each side of the bath bomb mold with a heaping amount of the bath salt mixture and then press tightly together. Any mixture that falls out and does not get pressed into the bath bomb should be put back into the bowl to press again.

5. Remove the bath bomb from the mold and place it on the tray with the parchment paper. After you have finished molding all the bath bombs, set the tray in a very dry area with good air circulation. Allow the bath bombs to dry for at least 12 hours.

6. After the bath bombs have dried, wrap them in cellophane with a silica moisture-absorbing packet and store for up to 3 months.

Fragrant Herbs Effervescent Rejuvenation Bath

This bath is mildly effervescent, which is achieved by reacting baking soda with rose hips. It uses a popular ingredient that I get a lot of formulation requests for—Epsom salt or Dead Sea salt—both of which contain a great deal of magnesium. Baths with this mineral will be relaxing as well as rejuvenating and pair perfectly with CBD infusion.

Makes about 32oz of effervescing bath salt

3 cups (560g) of Epsom salt or Dead Sea salt, fine grain

½ cup (115g) sodium bicarbonate (culinary baking soda)

½ cup (57g) soapwort root (Saponaria *officinalis*), powdered (no substitutions)

1 tbsp (15ml) or less CBD-infused camellia seed oil (page 22) (a concentrated, sifted hash-infused oil is suggested for best results with this recipe)

¼ cup (30g) rose hips, powdered

2 tablespoons, or a little more if desired, of dried aromatic herbs, powdered

1. Prepare a clean glass canning jar and new lid. Make sure this is very dry before starting.
2. In a glass or ceramic bowl, mix the Epsom or Dead Sea salt with the sodium bicarbonate and soapwort root until thoroughly combined. Add the CBD-infused camellia seed oil and work this into the salt mixture to distribute it evenly.
3. Add the powdered rose hip and any powdered aromatic herbs you would like to use to add fragrance to your bath salt. Work these ingredients thoroughly into the bath salt mixture until they are evenly distributed and have the fragrance you desire.
4. Scoop your finished bath salt into the glass canning jar with a silica moisture-absorbing packet and store for up to 3 months. Always use a clean and dry scoop to add this to your bath, and keep the jar tightly closed to prevent moisture from being absorbed by the magnesium-rich salts inside.

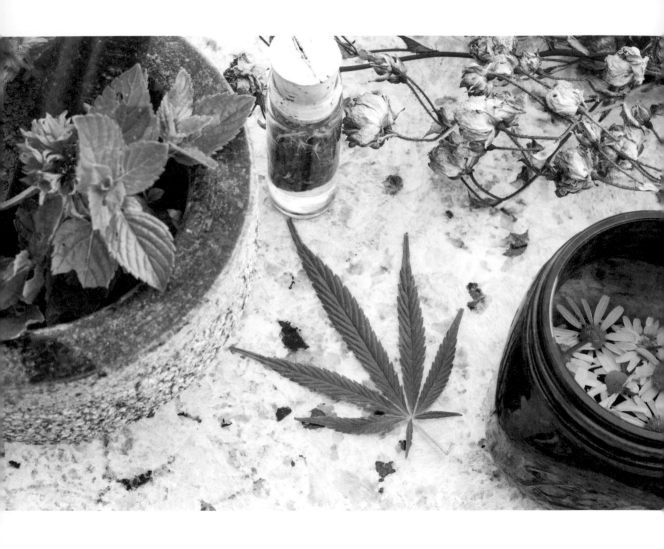

CHAPTER FOUR

CBD HERBAL APOTHECARY

Home remedies made with CBD are a popular way to enjoy the benefits of CBD. I've included some of my favorite home remedies here—but the best home remedies are the ones that you create! Many of the recipes in this chapter can be used as a basis for the herbs and flavors you would like to pair with CBD.

Lemon Mint Fever Frosty

A favorite creamy and cool beverage in my kitchen that I call a "frosty" for both its effervescence and cooling properties. I like this in the summer, or anytime I need relief from the heat of a fever or frequent hot flashes.

Makes approximately 2 (10 oz [600ml]) frosties

¾ cup (180ml) effervescent water (tepid room temperature)

⅓ cup (40g) powdered coconut milk

2 tsp (10ml) or less of CBD-infused coconut oil (page 25) (warmed to liquid state) or MCT oil (page 18)

½ cup (120ml) fresh-squeezed lemon juice, cold

½ cup (15g) fresh mint leaves

⅓ cup (80ml) honey, or more for sweeter frosties

2 cups (about 300ml) ice chips

1. Into the blender, pour the effervescent water first and then add the coconut milk powder and the warmed CBD oil. Blend until creamy and bubbly.
2. Add the lemon juice, mint leaves, honey, and ice chips to the liquid in the blender and blend until creamy. Serve immediately.

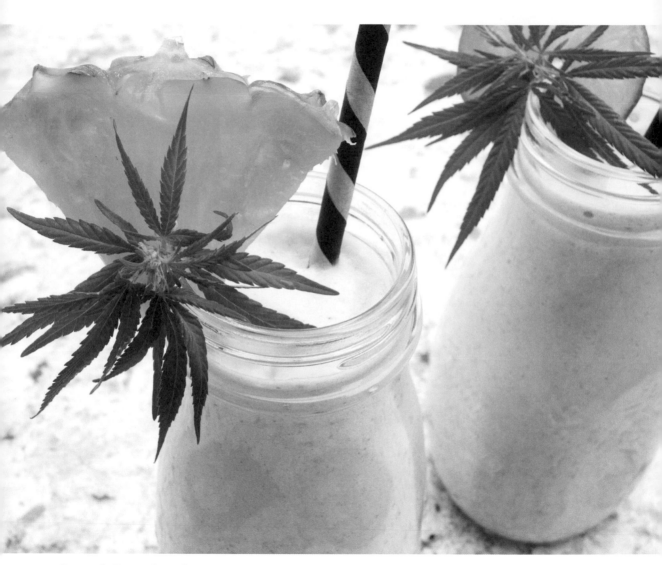

Pineapple Express Smoothie

Pineapple Express Smoothie

Unlock the enormous benefits of raw, juiced CBDA-rich cannabis in this delicious smoothie! Fresh CBDA-dominant cannabis flowers and leaves are a popular remedy and rich green vegetable without any psychoactive effects. When you use fresh cannabis, you actually incorporate the CBDA cannabinoid into whatever you are making—as long as heat is not applied, the end result will be CBDA—which has many of the same benefits as CBD, the decarboxylated molecule of CBDA.

You can make frozen cubes of blended, fresh CBDA-rich cannabis as described on page 36 and store them in your freezer as a handy way to make any smoothie or juice recipe. Or, use fresh clippings from any CBDA-dominant cannabis plant. Many people like to grow a small one on their windowsill to conveniently cut from for smoothies and juicing. A clone from a licensed dispensary is a good way to start doing this right away.

Makes approximately 2 (8 oz [480ml]) smoothies

1 whole pineapple, peeled, cored, and cut into slices
1 lime, juiced
¼ cup (60ml) ice chips
¼ cup (3–5g) living, CBDA-rich, cannabis flowers and leaves
Optional but amazing: 1 small whole jalapeño pepper

1. Peel, core, and slice the pineapple. Put the slices in the freezer for a few minutes to create a frostier smoothie. Cut the lime and squeeze the juice. Add this to the blender along with the ice chips.
2. Add the pineapple, cannabis, and the jalapeño pepper, if desired. Blend until rich and creamy.
3. Pour into glasses and garnish with pineapple slices, lime slices, and cannabis flowers. Serve immediately.

Mango Canna-Booster Smoothie

It's a well-known folk remedy in the medical cannabis community: boost the effects of cannabinoids by eating mangoes! I always recommend mangoes as a way to stretch your cannabis supply further. This smoothie is a great way to see if your personal CBD experience is enhanced with mango.

Makes approximately 2 (8oz [480ml]) smoothies

1. To a blender, add the coconut milk, CBD oil, and the orange juice. Blend until creamy.
2. Add the frozen mango slices and ice chips. Blend until icy and creamy. Serve immediately.

⅓ cup (40g) fresh coconut milk

2 tsp (10ml) or less CBD-infused coconut oil (page 25) (warmed to liquid state) or MCT oil (page 18)

1 cup (240ml) fresh-squeezed blood orange juice, room temperature (may substitute with any fresh-squeezed orange juice)

2 large or 3 medium mangoes, sliced and partially frozen

½ cup (about 100ml) ice chips

Ginger and Turmeric Hemp Smoothie

A quick and easy smoothie that will chase away morning aches and pains—guaranteed! This smoothie uses exclusively fresh ginger and turmeric; do not replace with dried, as the flavor will not be as bright and delicious.

Makes approximately 2 (8 oz [480ml]) smoothies

¾ cup (180ml) effervescent water (tepid room temperature)
¾ cup (130g) shelled hemp seeds
¼ tsp (0.25g) black pepper
2 tsp (10ml) or less CBD-infused coconut oil (page 25) or MCT oil (page 18)
2 thumb-sized pieces fresh ginger root, peeled
2 thumb-sized pieces fresh turmeric root, peeled
¼ cup (60ml) honey, or a little more to taste (However, this recipe can take any sweetener you desire, including sugar-free sweetener)
2 cups (about 300ml) ice chips

1. Into a blender, pour the effervescent water, hemp seeds, black pepper, and the CBD oil. Blend until creamy and bubbly.
2. Add the ginger, turmeric, honey or sweetener, and ice chips. Blend until smooth. Serve immediately.

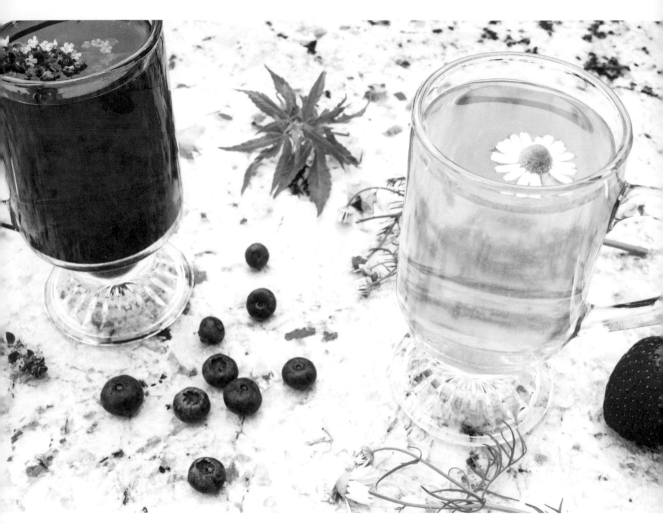

Effervescent Magnesium Cocktails

Effervescent Magnesium Cocktails

A bubbly and relaxing beverage that is an alternative to alcoholic beverages, these special CBD cocktails make the perfect beverage for happy hours, nightcaps, or celebratory occasions. In this beverage, CBD joins forces with magnesium to create the ultimate soothing relaxation without intoxicating effects.

The secret of this beverage is the combination of one sweet fruit and one herb that provide flavor and a foundation of naturally occurring terpenes as an entourage to maximize the benefits of CBD. Using this method of quick preparation to make the fresh fruit and herbs into a tisane with boiling water means they retain many of their raw benefits and vibrant, fresh flavors. Use the chart here to select the fruit and herb with the flavors and terpenes you desire, or create a combination of your own!

These warm magnesium cocktails are delicious, but be aware that consuming more than 1 to 2 teaspoons of magnesium supplement at one time may have laxative effects. Don't serve or consume more than two of these cocktails in a day. The typical suggested dose of CBD for this cocktail is around 25mg, but you can adjust this amount based on personal preferences.

Makes 2 (6 oz [180ml]) cocktails

½ cup, or more (60g–100g) of fruit

1 tbsp (3g) fresh herbs, or a little less if using dried herbs. Fresh is preferable to dried in this recipe.

2 tsp (2g) powdered magnesium supplement, packed (the label should state that this is a combination of citric acid and magnesium carbonate)

12oz (360ml) of boiling water

CBD beverage infusion with tincture (page 35)

1 tbsp (15ml) warm water

1. Rinse and prepare the desired fruit and fresh herbs. Place these in a pot or pan after they are prepared.

2. Prepare the serving cups by adding 1 teaspoon (1g) of magnesium into each of the cups.

3. Bring the water to a rolling boil. Pour the water into the pot or pan with the fruit and herbs. With a wooden pestle or spoon, smash the fruit and herbs to extract their juices into the hot water. After smashing, allow

this to sit for 5 minutes and then strain the fruit and herb liquid from the plant material.

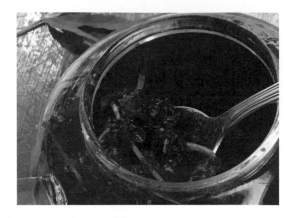

4. In a small bowl, combine the amount of CBD beverage infusion you desire for two servings of this cocktail (as described in the beverage infusion recipe on page 35) with the warm water and stir to dissolve. Take ½ cup (120ml) of the fruit-infused hot water and add it to this mixture. Whisk thoroughly. Pour this into the pot or pan with the rest of the hot fruit-infused water and whisk again to thoroughly combine.

5. Heat the liquid again on the stove until hot but not boiling. Whisk thoroughly. Remove from the heat.

6. Pour the hot liquid evenly into each cup and briefly stir. Garnish with a piece of fruit or herb and serve immediately to retain effervescence.

Fruit and Herb Pairing Chart

FRUIT	HERB	TERPENES
Blueberry	Lemon Thyme or Garden Thyme	Limonene, Citral, Myrcene, Caryophyllene
Strawberry	Chamomile	Bisabolol, Chamazulene, Myrcene
Pineapple	Rosemary	Caryophyllene, Pinene, Linalool, Limonene, Myrcene
Orange (pith and peel removed)	Lavender	Limonene, Linalool, Citral, Terpineol, Linalyl acetate
Apple	Spearmint	Carvone, Farnesene, Limonene, Pinene, Cineol
Peach	Basil	Eugenol, Limonene, Ionone, Linalool, Cinnamate, Myrcene

Maiden and Crone Elixirs

Both of these elixirs contain one of my favorite herbs: angelica root, otherwise known as dong quai in Chinese medicine. It's a versatile herb, one used both for folk remedy decoctions or elixirs, and is also used in broth and soup recipes. It's excellent in chicken broth and has a very strong celery flavor, as it is related to the celery plant. However, in decoctions or elixirs, it is quite medicinal tasting—an acquired taste, if you will. The Crone elixir has been so helpful for my hot flashes that come with menopause that it's a welcome flavor. I've also been told that the Maiden elixir was quite effective for the aches and pains that come with PMS, bloating, and period cramps! Try it and see what you think. Do not use this elixir if you are pregnant, nursing, or trying to get pregnant.

Makes 2 or more elixirs

The instructions are the same for both maiden and crone versions of this recipe.

For the Maiden Elixir:
CBD beverage infusion with tincture (page 35)
3 cups (720ml) water + more if needed through the boiling process
2 large slices angelica root, dried
¼ cup (20g) peony root (Paeonia lactiflora), dried
¼ cup (15g) goji berry
10 large red jujube dates

For the Crone Elixir:
CBD beverage infusion with tincture (page 35) 3 cups (720 ml) water + more if needed through the boiling process
2 large slices angelica root, dried
10 large red jujube dates

1. Select and measure the right amount of CBD beverage infusion with tincture (page 35) that you desire to use with this elixir. Set aside.
2. In a ceramic or glass cooking vessel, such as a glass teapot, add the water and all the ingredients, except for the CBD beverage infusion tincture.
3. Turn on the stove to medium and simmer for 45 minutes. Add more water during the simmer process if you want a less concentrated elixir. The ingredients as listed here make at least 2 or more servings of elixir.
4. Remove from the heat and pour the liquid through a tea strainer into a serving pot. Add the CBD beverage tincture mixture and whisk thoroughly into the elixir. Pour the desired amount of elixir into cups and serve. Any leftover elixir can be stored in a glass canning jar in the refrigerator and is good if used within 3 days. Warm the elixir again before serving.

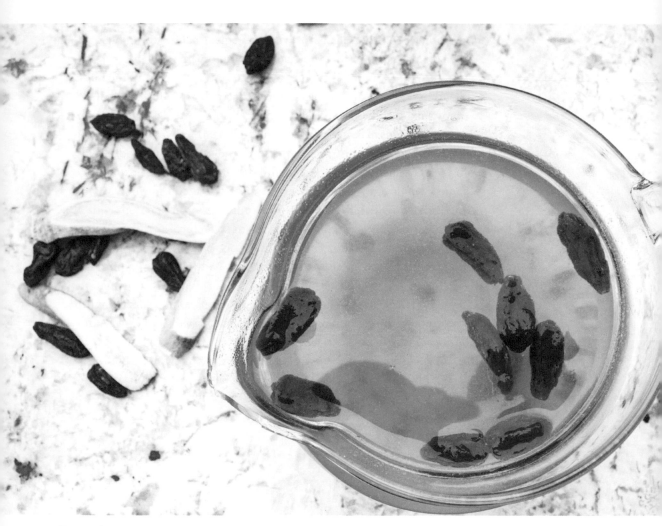

Forest Elixir

Forest Elixir

The benefits and nourishment that come from the beloved white pine tree have been known to foragers for centuries. Pine needles are rich in vitamin C, and pine resin is rich in powerful terpenes that are renowned for soothing sore throats. This recipe uses foraged ingredients. Pine trees are easy to find and harvesting their needles and resin is a simple process. Most pine trees will have some visible, dried resin that can be gently scraped off the tree without damaging the bark. Select the cleanest resin that has dried on the trunk of the tree for best results in this recipe.

Makes 2 or more elixirs

Cured and dried CBD-rich cannabis flowers and leaves, decarboxylated (page 31)
3 cups (720ml) water
1 cup (30g) fresh white pine needles
1 tbsp (10g) white pine resin
1 cut lemon to garnish or squeeze

1. Select and measure the amount of CBD-rich cannabis plant material in the dosage size you desire. In a ceramic or glass cooking vessel, such as a glass teapot, add all the ingredients, including the cannabis.
2. On medium heat, simmer everything for 30 minutes. Remove from the stove and pour through a tea strainer into cups. Leftover elixir can be kept in the refrigerator for up to 3 days and reheated again. Garnish with a slice of cut lemon to squeeze into the elixir and serve immediately.

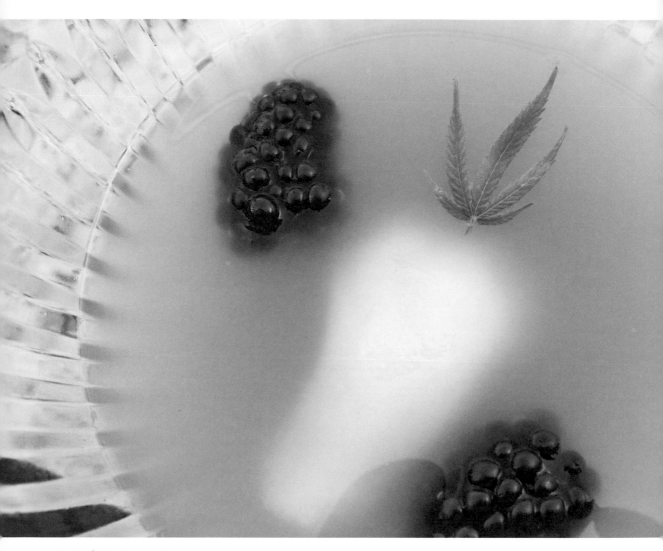

Revitalizing Dessert Soup

Revitalizing Dessert Soup

Fruit soups are a refreshing way to revitalize both your mood and your body. My favorite recipe for fruit soup infused with CBD tincture is one made with the Himalayan blackberry, a local and invasive (but very tasty) wild blackberry. Fresh-pressed apple cider is suggested for this recipe.

Makes 2–4 servings

4 cups (1L) fresh-pressed apple cider
1 large thumb-sized piece fresh ginger, peeled
2 fresh, large pears, peeled and sliced into halves
24 fresh blackberries
CBD beverage infusion with tincture (page 35)
1 tbsp (15ml) warm water
Several fresh mint leaves and sprigs

1. In a blender, add 1 cup (240ml) of the apple cider and ginger. Blend until smooth. Add the rest of the apple cider and blend thoroughly.
1. In a pan on the stove, add the apple cider infused with ginger and the pear halves. Cover and simmer on medium-low for 20 to 30 minutes or until the pears are soft.
2. Add the whole blackberries and cover once again and simmer for 1 minute. Remove from the heat.
3. In a small bowl, combine the amount of CBD tincture that you desire for 4 servings of this soup (as described in the beverage infusion recipe on page 35) with the water. Take ½ cup (120ml) of just liquid from the soup pan and add it to this mixture. Whisk thoroughly.
4. Pour the liquid infused with CBD that you have just made back into the pan of hot soup and combine thoroughly without breaking or mashing the fruit. Pour the hot fruit soup into bowls immediately, serving one pear half per bowl. Garnish with several mint sprigs on top of the soup for flavor and presentation. Serve immediately.

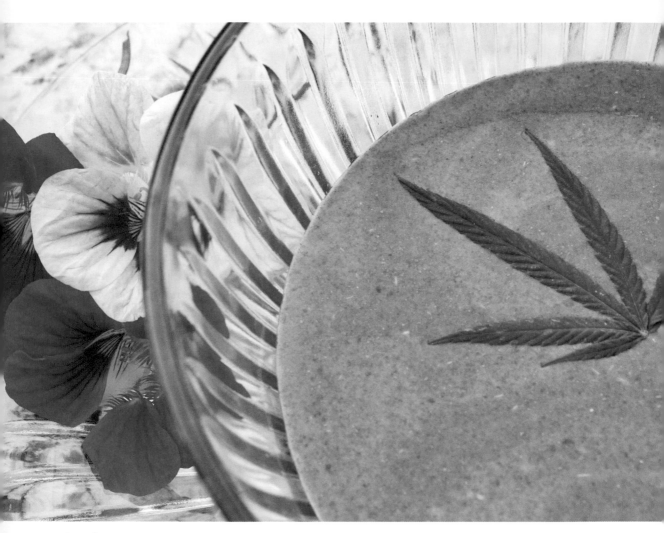

Spiced Lime Moringa Soup

Spiced Lime Moringa Soup

This is a nourishing and warming CBD-infused soup best prepared in a blender with a soup setting. Alternatively, this may be gently warmed on the stove and then served immediately.

Makes approximately 2 (8oz [480ml]) cups of soup

2 cups (480ml) fresh coconut milk

2 tsp (10ml) or less CBD-infused coconut oil (page 25) or MCT oil (page 18)

1 thumb-sized piece fresh ginger, peeled

1 large lime, fresh juice only

1 or more fresh Thai peppers

1 small clove garlic

¼ cup (25g) moringa powder

Sea salt to taste

Cracked white peppercorn to taste

Thin slices of lime for garnish

1. Add the coconut milk and CBD oil to the blender and blend thoroughly.
2. Add the rest of the ingredients, including the salt and pepper. Set the blender to the soup setting and blend until warm and creamy. Otherwise, transfer to a pan on the stove after the soup has blended and warm gently before serving.
3. Garnish with a thin slice of lime and serve immediately.

Winter Blues Herbal Broth

This is a simple vegetable broth that infuses CBD into a winter blues–busting broth that uses whatever leftover vegetables you have in your kitchen, along with blueberries, ginger, lemon, and the precious seasoning blend known as Herbes de Provence. Enjoy on a snow day!

Makes 2–4 servings

1. In a blender, combine the water and all the fresh-cut fruit and vegetables—do not add the sliced lemon or additional blueberries. Blend until chopped. Transfer the mixture to a pan on the stove. Now you can add the whole lemon slices.
2. Cover the pan and set the heat to medium. Simmer for 60 minutes, or until all the chopped ingredients have turned to mush and released their juices. Simmer for another 15 minutes with the lid off the pan to allow the liquid to reduce and concentrate more flavor.
3. Remove from the stove and pour through a strainer and cheesecloth into another pan on the stove. Squeeze as much of the vegetable juice out as you can using the cheesecloth.
4. In a cup, combine the amount of CBD tincture that you desire for 4 servings of this soup (as described in the beverage infusion recipe on page 35) with the water. Take ½ cup (120ml) of the strained broth and add it to this mixture. Whisk thoroughly.
5. Pour the liquid infused with CBD that you have just made back into the pan of hot broth and combine thoroughly.
6. Salt and pepper to taste and add the Herbes de Provence. Add the additional whole blueberries and heat on medium-low, covered, for 10 minutes. Remove from the stove and taste again. Adjust salt and pepper as desired. Pour into bowls and serve immediately.

4 cups (1L) water
fresh cut vegetable and fruit mix: 5 medium carrots, 2 medium celery stalks, 1 pepper, 1 onion, 3 large tomatoes, 3 large cloves garlic, 1 large thumb-sized piece ginger, 12 blueberries
1 lemon, sliced into thin slices
CBD beverage infusion with tincture (page 35)
Cracked black pepper to taste and sea salt
1 tsp (1g) dried herb mix of Herbes de Provence (these are typically thyme, rosemary, lavender, savory, marjoram)
1 tbsp (15ml) warm water
12 additional blueberries

The Essential Tinctures

My personal CBD medicine cabinet generally has one or more of these four tinctures available at any time. CBD or CBDA can be infused into these tinctures along with the other herbs, depending on your preference. As a general rule of thumb, I do think that tinctures work best when there is at least 5mg to 10mg of CBD or CBDA per 1ml serving. The amount of CBD or CBDA-rich cannabis that you add should be based on the calculations you have made for each serving size you desire.

Quick Relief Tincture

A simple formula for pain relief that pairs the anti-inflammatory roots of peony with CBD cannabis and other inflammation-fighting herbs.

Makes about 4oz (120ml) tincture

¼ cup (25g) peony root, dried and sliced

2 tbsp (15g) frankincense serrata resin

2 large thumb-sized pieces fresh ginger root, peeled and chopped

CBD-rich cured cannabis flowers (decarboxylated before tincturing page 31), or CBDA-rich cured cannabis flowers

½ cup (120ml) 150-proof culinary alcohol (or a little more as needed to cover the herbs)

1. Put all the herbs, including the cannabis, into an amber glass canning jar. Pour the alcohol over them. The alcohol should cover all the herbs completely. Affix the lid.
2. Prepare a pan with very warm water and allow the jar to sit in the warm water until it cools to room temperature. This step will soften the resins and other ingredients. Shake the jar and put in a dark, warm spot in the kitchen.
3. Allow the jar to rest for 3 to 4 weeks for best results. Shake the jar at least twice a week.
4. Shake the jar before decanting and straining the tincture from the herbs through cheesecloth lining a strainer. Squeeze out as much of the liquid from the herbs as possible.
5. Prepare clean glass tincture bottles with dropper caps. Using a funnel or spout, fill each bottle and affix the caps. Use within 6 months for best results.

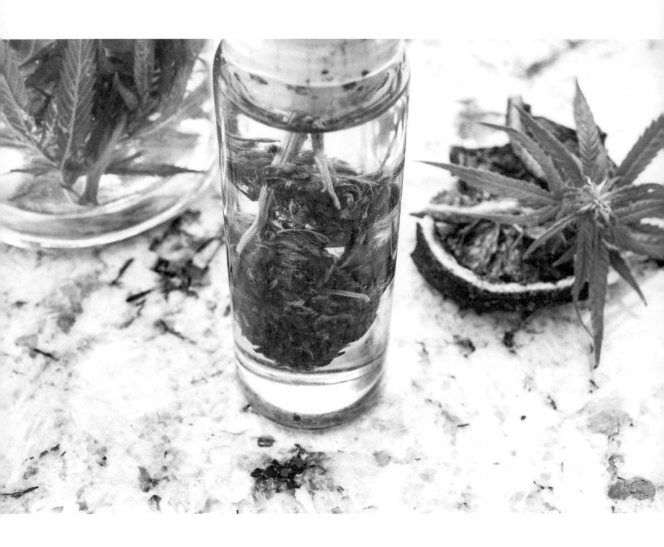

Sleepy-Time Tincture

A relaxing blend of herbs paired with CBD-rich cannabis. Try this in hot water or hot lemon balm tea before bed.

Makes about 4oz (120ml) tincture

2 large thumb-sized pieces fresh turmeric, chopped
¼ cup (15g) fresh or dried chamomile flowers
¼ cup (15g) fresh or dried lemon balm leaves
½ tsp (1g) whole black peppercorns
CBD-rich cured cannabis flowers (decarboxylated before tincturing page 31), or CBDA-rich cured cannabis flowers
½ cup (120ml) 150-proof culinary alcohol (or a little more as needed to cover the herbs)

1. Put all the herbs, including the cannabis, into an amber glass canning jar. Pour the alcohol over them. The alcohol should cover all the herbs completely. Affix the lid.

2. Prepare a pan with very warm water and allow the jar to sit in the warm water until it cools to room temperature. This step will soften the resins and other ingredients. Shake the jar and put in a dark, warm spot in the kitchen.

3. Allow the jar to rest for 3 to 4 weeks for best results. Shake the jar at least twice a week.

4. Shake the jar before decanting and straining the tincture from the herbs through cheesecloth lining a strainer. Squeeze out as much of the liquid from the herbs as possible.

5. Prepare clean glass tincture bottles with dropper caps. Using a funnel or spout, fill each bottle and affix the caps. Use within 6 months for best results.

Mood Therapy Tincture

This is an extremely effective mood-lifting tincture infused with CBD that's great for when you are having a bad day or just feeling a little blue.

Makes about 4oz (120ml) tincture

1. Put all the herbs, including the cannabis, into an amber glass canning jar. Pour the alcohol over them. The alcohol should cover all the herbs completely. Affix the lid.
2. Prepare a pan with very warm water and allow the jar to sit in the warm water until it cools to room temperature. This step will soften the resins and other ingredients. Shake the jar and put in a dark, warm spot in the kitchen.
3. Allow the jar to rest for 3 to 4 weeks for best results. Shake the jar at least twice a week.
4. Shake the jar before decanting and straining the tincture from the herbs through cheesecloth lining a strainer. Squeeze out as much of the liquid from the herbs as possible.
5. Prepare clean glass tincture bottles with dropper caps. Using a funnel or spout, fill each bottle and affix the caps. Use within 6 months for best results.

⅓ cup or 5 sprigs (18g) fresh rosemary
1 tbsp (6g) ashwagandha powder
50 saffron threads
1 tbsp (8g) frankincense serrata resin
CBD-rich cured cannabis flowers (decarboxylated before tincturing page 31), or CBDA-rich cured cannabis flowers
½ cup (120ml) 150-proof culinary alcohol (or a little more as needed to cover the herbs)

Detox Tincture

Detox means a bunch of different things to many people. In my herbal remedy repertoire "detox" is a kind of bitters tincture to have around when you've had a little too much to eat or drink. Cannabis is a bitter and cooling herb and since this tincture is infused with bitter herbs and CBD-rich cannabis, you'll feel the relief right away.

Makes about 4oz (120ml) tincture

1 medium-sized fresh burdock root, chopped
1 medium orange, peels only, chopped (wash the orange to remove any coatings before using in this recipe)
1 medium fresh dandelion root, washed, peeled, chopped
1 tsp (2g) fennel seeds
1 tbsp (8g) milk thistle
CBD-rich cured cannabis flowers (decarboxylated before tincturing page 31), or CBDA-rich cured cannabis flowers
½ cup (120ml) 150-proof culinary alcohol (or a little more as needed to cover the herbs)

1. Put all the herbs, including the cannabis, into an amber glass canning jar. Pour the alcohol over them. The alcohol should cover all the herbs completely. Affix the lid.
2. Prepare a pan with very warm water and allow the jar to sit in the warm water until it cools to room temperature. This step will soften the resins and other ingredients. Shake the jar and put in a dark, warm spot in the kitchen.
3. Allow the jar to rest for 3 to 4 weeks for best results. Shake the jar at least twice a week.
4. Shake the jar before decanting and straining the tincture from the herbs through cheesecloth lining a strainer. Squeeze out as much of the liquid from the herbs as possible.
5. Prepare clean glass tincture bottles with dropper caps. Using a funnel or spout, fill each bottle and affix the caps. Use within 6 months for best results.

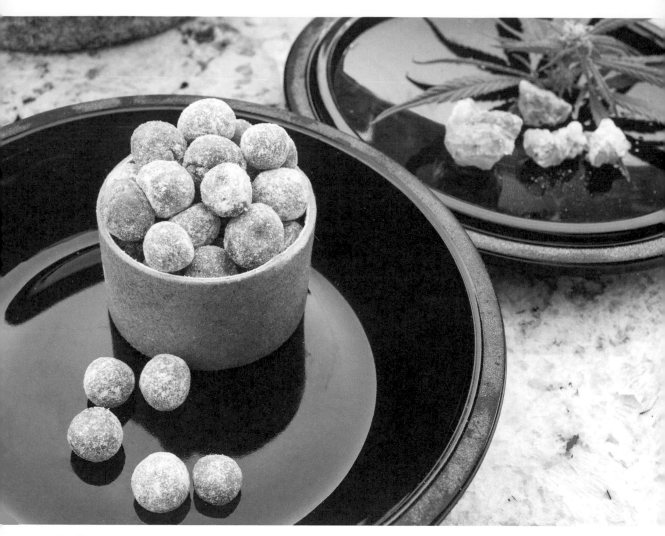

"Roll Your Own" Pain Pills

"Roll Your Own" Pain Pills

Everyone loves pain pills. More pain-relieving pharmaceutical drugs are sold in the USA than any other class of drug. From prescription-only opioid pain relievers like Oxycontin and fentanyl to the over-the-counter drugs like ibuprofen and Tylenol—we love our pharmaceutical pain pills. And we love them to death.[12] People die because these pills become a life-style—instead of a rare necessity.

There are many of us who have rejected the death culture of pharmaceutical pain pills and have taken back our liberty to manage own own pain with home remedies. In locations where cannabis—CBD and all other cannabinoids—are legal, this gentle herb is often included in home remedies for pain management.

Pain pills are loved by humans for the convenience and ofen fast relief they offer. When your hips and knees ache, the last thing you want to do is stand on your feet and make a decoction. We all want to lie down and pop some pain pills.

Now, if you've ever tried to make herbal gel capsules at home, you know how difficult they are to fill, the tendency to leak and get sticky, and sometimes they are a challenge to swallow. This recipe uses the ancient pill-making technique of rolling small (pea-size or smaller) spherical "pills" from a dough of blended herbs, resins, and oils. Because you are "rolling your own," these pills can be made as small as you need to make them—unlike gel capsules that have standard sizes and aren't always suitable for people who need very small pills to swallow comfortably.

This easy-to-make pain pill recipe is made with simple ingredients and infused with measured doses of CBD so you can conveniently pop these whenever you need to. CBD pairs with a base of either pure frankincense

---

12 Annual Causes of Death in the United States, https://www.drugwarfacts.org/chapter/causes_of_death.

serrata or frankincense frereana—both of which are noted in traditional folk medicine practices of India and the Middle East for managing pain and inflammation while being cooling and soothing for the stomach. This recipe uses whole resin only; purchasing this resin in the powdered form is the most convenient way to work with this recipe. Do not replace whole resin frankincense with essential oil of frankincense—they are not the same.

Create your pills using the concentration of CBD you have calculated for each pill. I've had great results making these pills with 3mg to 5mg of CBD per pill and taking as many as 5 pills at a time. For proper digestion, always take 1 at a time if you are taking more than 1, and always drink a glass of water.

Makes 100 or more small pea-sized "pills" or smaller

1. In a bowl, combine the frankincense powder and acacia gum. Add the CBD oil and combine with the dry ingredients until it is thoroughly distributed.
2. Add the boiling water and stir and knead until you have a "dough." Add a little arrowroot powder as needed to bring this together so that it is not sticky and can be easily rolled between your fingers.
3. Begin to roll out the pills in pea-sized pieces or smaller. Coat them in a little arrowroot powder as they are rolled.
4. Place the pills on parchment paper on the drying rack of a dehydrator or in a slightly warm oven on a tray and allow them to dry at very low temperatures. The ideal drying temperature is 120° F (48° C) or less, and they will take about 2 to 6 hours to completely dry depending on the environment.

½ cup (60g) whole food-grade frankincense serrata or frankincense frereana resin, powdered

2 tbsp (15g) acacia gum, powdered

2 tbsp (30ml) CBD-infused coconut oil, melted (concentrated with the dosage you desire for each pill on page 25)

2 tsp (10ml) boiling water, or a little more as needed to bring the other ingredients together into a pliable dough

Arrowroot, powdered

5. Alternatively, the dough may be worked into a silicone mold with your desired "pill" sizes. This can be dried at low temperatures as described in step 4. When the pills are easily popped from the mold, put them on parchment paper and continue following the instructions in step 4 and complete their drying cycle

6. When the pills are dry, allow them to cool completely and transfer to the containers you would like to store them in. Amber glass bottles are suggested for best shelf life. Always store the pills with silica moisture-absorbing packets made for food storage. This is a must that you should not skip; the gums are very prone to picking up moisture from the environment. Use the pills within 6 months for best results.

Herbal Pills for What Ails You

This is another great "pill" you can make in your own kitchen—and it happens to be the "Swiss army knife" of CBD remedies! Three great plant ingredients (myrrh, ashwagandha, and CBD) synergize together to bring symptom relief any time of the day. For proper digestion, alway take 1 at a time if you are taking more than 1, and always drink a glass of water.

Makes 100 or more small pea-sized "'pills'" or smaller

1. In a bowl combine the myrrh powder, acacia gum, and ashwagandha powder. Add the CBD oil and stir until it is evenly distributed throughout the dry mixture.
2. Add the boiling water and stir and knead until you have a dough. Add a little arrowroot powder as needed to bring this together so that it is not sticky and can be easily rolled between your fingers.
3. Begin to roll out the pills in pea-sized pieces or smaller. Coat them in a little arrowroot powder as they are rolled.
4. Place the pills on parchment paper on the drying rack of a dehydrator or in a slightly warm oven on a tray and allow them to dry at very low temperatures. The ideal drying temperature is 120° F (48° C) or less, and they will take about 2 to 6 hours to completely dry depending on the environment.
5. Alternatively, the dough may be worked into a silicone mold with your desired "pill" sizes. This can be dried at low temperatures as described in step 4. When the pills are easily popped from the mold, put them on parchment paper and continue following the instructions in step 4 and complete their drying cycle

¼ cup (30g) powdered food-grade myrrh gum

2 tbsp (15g) acacia gum, powdered

¼ cup (25g) ashwagandha powder

2 tbsp (30ml) CBD-infused coconut oil, melted (concentrated with the dosage you desire for each pill on page 25)

1 tbsp (15ml) boiling water, or a little more as needed to bring the other ingredients together into a pliable dough

arrowroot, powdered

6. When the pills are dry, allow them to cool completely and transfer to the containers you would like to store them in. Amber glass bottles are suggested for best shelf life. Always store the pills with silica moisture-absorbing packets made for food storage. This is a must that you should not skip, as the gums are very prone to picking up moisture from the environment. Use the pills within 6 months for best results.

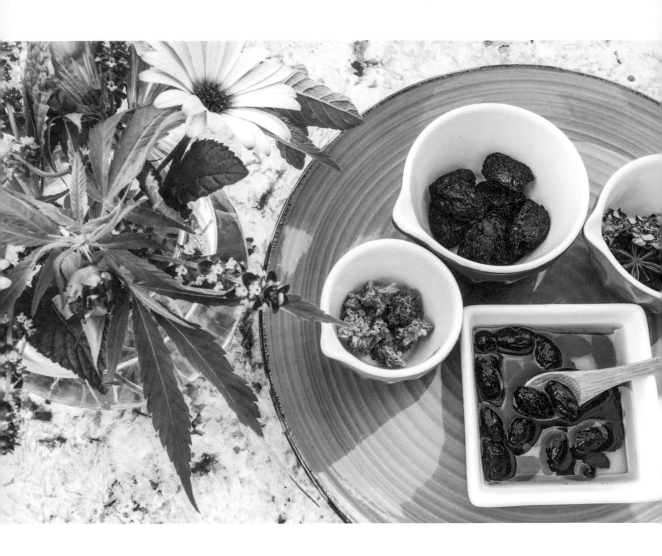

CHAPTER FIVE

CBD SWEET AND SAVORY FOR YOU AND YOUR GUESTS

CBD makes a fantastic culinary ingredient—especially if you would like to create a relaxing but completely sober experience for yourself or guests. CBD is also an excellent way to balance the effects of THC-infused food and beverages so that the effects are gentler. Using CBD in this way is similar to the experience one would have while enjoying moderate amounts of wine in a dining or wine hour event.

The recipes in this chapter are versatile and will serve many different guests—free of all eight major allergens (soy, dairy, egg, wheat [gluten], shellfish, fish, peanut, tree nut), there is something for everyone!

The Sweet

Bhang is a creamy cannabis-infused beverage that has been enjoyed in India and the rest of southern Asia for thousands of years. There are many different recipes and ways to prepare this beverage; these two recipes are infused with CBD-rich cannabis and fresh fruit for a creamy beverage that is both delicious and satisfying.

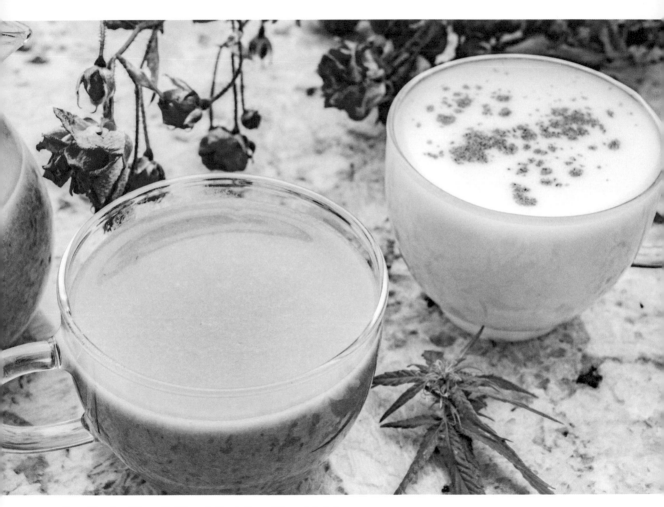

Rose Garden Bhang (left) and *Fresh Pear Bhang* (right)

Fresh Pear Bhang

Makes 2 or more servings

1 large pear, peeled, cored, sliced
1½ cups (360ml) fresh coconut milk
1 tsp (5ml) vanilla extract
1 tsp (5ml) or less CBD-infused coconut oil (page 25)
Any sweetener as desired
Pinch of shaved nutmeg to dust the top of each cup of bhang

1. To a blender, add the pear, coconut milk, and the vanilla extract. Blend until creamy and smooth. Transfer the liquid to a pan on the stove.
2. Place the pan of bhang over medium heat until it simmers. Add the CBD-infused coconut oil and sweetener as desired. Continue to simmer for 2 more minutes while whisking.
3. Pour into cups, dust nutmeg shavings over the top, and serve immediately.

Rose Garden Bhang

Makes 2 or more servings

¼ cup (40g) raspberries
1 tbsp (15ml) culinary rose water
1½ cups (360ml) fresh coconut milk
1 tsp (5ml) vanilla extract
1 tsp (5ml) or less CBD-infused coconut oil (page 25)
Any sweetener as desired
Whole raspberries to garnish each cup of bhang

1. To a blender, add the raspberries, rose water, coconut milk, and vanilla extract. Blend until creamy and smooth. Transfer the liquid to a pan on the stove.
2. Place the pan of bhang over medium heat until it simmers. Add the CBD-infused coconut oil, and sweetener as desired. Continue to simmer for 2 more minutes while whisking.
3. Pour into cups, garnish with fresh raspberries, and serve immediately.

Shortbread Cookies

A delightful gluten and big-eight allergen-free shortbread cookie infused with CBD—perfect for many occasions and guests. Two recipes in one: lemon lavender and raspberry white chocolate!

Makes about 24 cookies

Special tools for this recipe:
A decorative cookie press for molding cookies solid before baking

Dry Base Ingredients:
1 cup (120g) sweet white rice flour
½ cup (65g) sorghum flour
¾ cup (160g) sugar
¼ cup (40g) millet flour
1 tbsp (8g) arrowroot flour
1 tsp (2.5g) acacia gum powder
½ tsp (2.5g) baking powder
½ tsp (3g) salt
½ tsp (3g) black salt (kala namak)

For the Lavender Lemon Shortbread:
2 tsp (10ml) vanilla extract
2 tsp (10ml) white bean or chickpea aquafaba
1 tsp (1g) lavender flowers
2 tsp (2g) grated lemon zest
½ cup (120ml) melted coconut oil infused with CBD (from page 25)

For the White Chocolate Raspberry Shortbread:
2 tsp (10ml) vanilla extract
2 tsp (10ml) white bean or chickpea aquafaba
¼ cup (8g) of freeze-dried raspberries, crushed into small pieces
½ cup (120ml) melted cacao butter infused with CBD (from page 25)

1. Preheat the oven to 350° F (177° C). Prepare a silicone baking sheet or line a baking sheet with parchment paper.
2. In a bowl, combine all the dry base ingredients thoroughly. Select either the Lavender Lemon or the White Chocolate Raspberry cookie ingredients and measure.

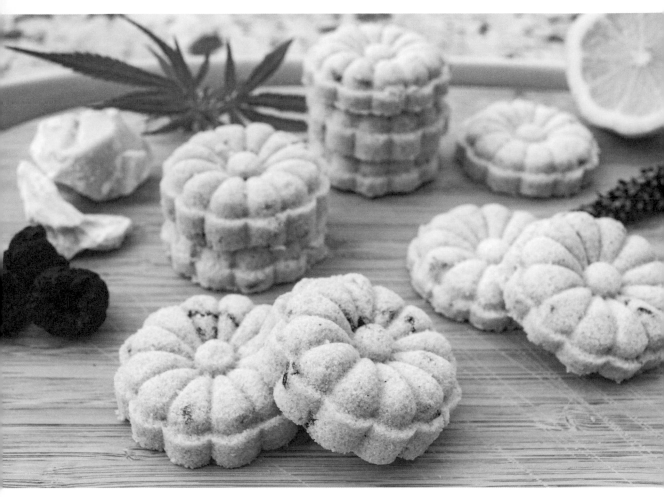

Shortbread Cookies

3. Combine the vanilla extract and aquafaba together in a cup. Add to the dry mixture and combine thoroughly to distribute evenly throughout the mixture.

4. Depending on which recipe you have selected, add the lavender and lemon zest or the freeze-dried raspberries to the dry base ingredients and combine.

5. Melt the CBD-infused coconut oil or cacao butter before adding to the other ingredients. Add the melted oil or butter while mixing to distribute evenly, When the oil or butter is distributed evenly, the mixture should be about the same texture as wet sand and easily press together.

6. On a surface covered with parchment paper, spoon out some of the mixture into a pile and flatten down to a little more than ½ inch. Using the cookie press, stamp down on the flattened mixture and press to form a cookie. Transfer to the baking sheet, and continue until all the mixture has been shaped into cookies. Each cookie will be approximately ½ inch high and about 1½ inches or a little more in diameter.

7. After all the cookies are on the baking sheet, bake at 350° F (177° C) for 15 minutes. Remove from the oven and allow to cool completely before serving or moving. As these cookies are gluten-free, to prevent crumbling, always cool completely before serving or storing.

8. Store for up to a week in an airtight container.

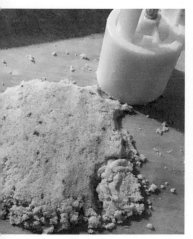
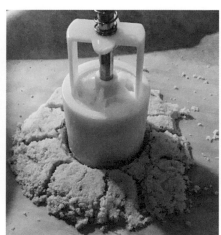
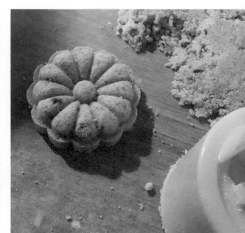

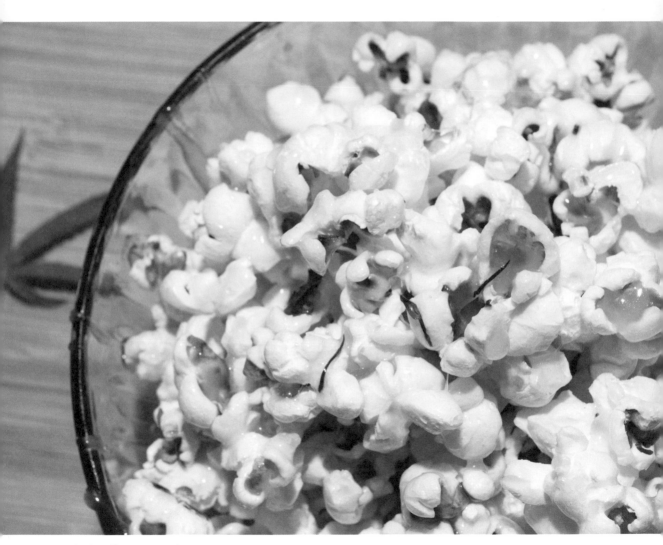

Salted Saffron Caramel Popcorn

Salted Saffron Caramel Popcorn

This coconut-based CBD- and saffron-infused caramel turns popcorn into an elegant treat that you can serve for occasions like the holidays or just to treat yourself to something sweet and special.

Makes several servings

¾ cup (180ml) fresh coconut milk

25 saffron threads

2 tsp (15ml) vanilla extract

1 cup (200g) unbleached cane sugar

1 tsp (6g) sea salt or smoked salt

1 tbsp (15ml) CBD-infused coconut oil (page 25)

⅓ cup (100g) or more popcorn kernels (about 10 cups finished popcorn), popped in coconut oil or air popped, and salted to taste

1. In a pan on the stove, gently warm, but do not steam, the coconut milk, saffron threads, and vanilla extract. Remove from the stove and allow the saffron to release all of the color and flavor into the coconut milk, about 20 minutes or so.

2. Return the pan to the stove and add the sugar and the sea salt to the coconut milk and dissolve completely on low heat. Turn the heat up to medium-high and attach a candy thermometer inside the pan. Stir and allow the mixture to reach 270° F (132° C). Remove from the heat and stir in the CBD oil immediately.

3. Spread the popped and salted popcorn on a baking sheet lined with parchment. Drizzle the hot caramel sauce over the popcorn. Allow it to rest for a minute or more until you can form into popcorn balls, if you desire. Otherwise it can be left to set up in a cool area or in the refrigerator for a few minutes and then spooned into a bowl for serving. The popcorn will keep in an airtight container for up to 5 days for the best flavor.

4. Leftover caramel can be kept in the refrigerator and re-softened by adding a little water and reheating on the stove on low heat.

Gooey Brownie Pie

A decadent brownie pie like this is the perfect way to infuse CBD! This is easy to make and bakes quickly to perfection with a nice crunchy crust and gooey inside.

Makes 1 standard 8-inch (20cm) pie pan

1. Preheat the oven to 425° F (218° C). Prepare a pie pan by greasing and dusting with some flour, or use a silicone pie pan.
2. In a mixing bowl, combine the flour, cacao, sugar, salt, kala namak, baking powder, and coconut milk powder thoroughly.
3. In a small bowl combine the aquafaba, vanilla extract, and CBD oil. Stir until combined and smooth.
4. Pour the liquid ingredients into the dry ingredients while mixing. Once this is thoroughly combined, pour it into the pie pan and put it into the oven. Bake until the outside is crispy, but the inside is hot and gooey, roughly 15 minutes. Remove from the oven.
5. Dust the top with a little powdered sugar. The pie can be served immediately. This gooey pie is great when topped with ice cream too!

1½ cups (190g) any gluten-free grain flour blend
½ cup (70g) raw cacao powder
1 cup (200g) unbleached cane sugar
½ tsp (3g) sea salt
Pinch of (black salt) kala namak
1½ tsp (7g) baking powder
½ cup (75g) powdered coconut milk
1 cup (240ml) white bean or chickpea aquafaba
1 tbsp (15ml) vanilla extract
3 tbsp (45ml) CBD-infused coconut oil (page 25), melted
Powdered sugar for dusting

Arkansas Black Apple Cake

The Arkansas black apple came to my attention after medicinal cannabis was legalized in Arkansas. It's an old-fashioned country apple that has been cultivated since the nineteenth century with unique color and flavor that changes from tart to sweet after harvesting. It's known as a "black apple" for its deep burgundy color, which becomes more intense during storage. (These apples can be stored for three months or a little more after picking.) I like these apples when they are freshly picked and very tart. They make an excellent CBD-infused apple cake with lush apple flavor that's a little tart and a little sweet.

This cake is made with coconut oil that has been infused with CBD-rich cannabis flowers. You can infuse any form of CBD you have on hand into coconut oil—the oil in this cake should be prepared before making this cake.

Makes one 8-inch x 8-inch (20cm x 20cm) square cake

1½ cups (270g) sweet brown rice flour
¾ cup (120g) millet flour
1 cup (220g) sugar
½ cup (60g) arrowroot flour
1 tbsp (12g) baking powder
2 tsp (4g) ginger powder
1 tsp (2g) cinnamon
1½ tsp (4g) acacia gum powder
½ tsp (1g) allspice powder
1 tsp (6g) sea salt
½ cup (120ml) CBD-infused coconut oil, melted
2 tbsp (30ml) water
½ cup (120ml) white bean or chickpea aquafaba

For the apple topping:
Juice of 1 medium-sized lemon
2–3 sliced Arkansas black apples (or substitute any apple, but these are the best)
1 tbsp (7g) arrowroot powder
1 tbsp (15g) sugar
½ tsp (1g) cinnamon
1 tbsp (15ml) CBD-infused coconut oil, melted

1. Preheat the oven to 350° F (177° C). Prepare the baking pan that you will be using. If the pan is silicone or nonstick, do not grease. If the pan is not nonstick, grease with a little coconut oil and flour the surface with a little arrowroot powder after greasing and set aside.
2. In a bowl, combine all the dry ingredients first: rice flour, millet flour, sugar, arrowroot, baking powder, ginger, cinnamon, acacia gum, allspice, and sea salt. Set aside.
3. Juice the lemon. Peel and core the apples. Slice lengthwise into thin slices that can be arranged neatly on top of the cake. Immediately toss them with the juice of the lemon to prevent browning.
4. In a ziptop bag, combine the arrowroot powder, sugar, and cinnamon. Drain the lemon juice from the apples. Add the tablespoon of

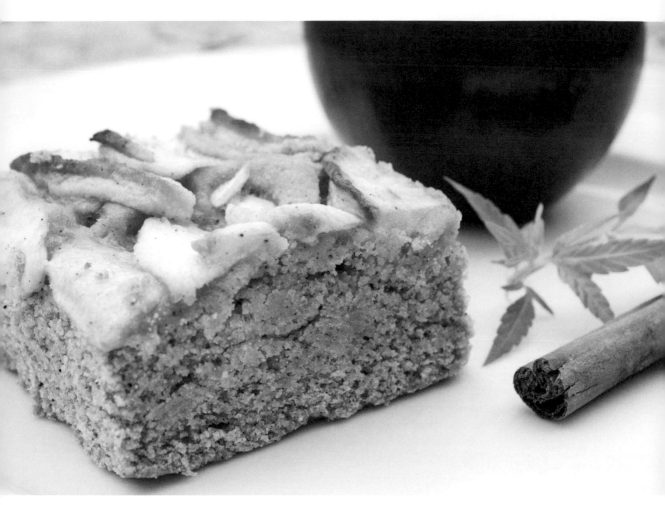

Arkansas Black Apple Cake

CBD-infused coconut oil to the apples and toss to coat with the oil. Spoon them into the bag and shake to coat with the dry ingredients. Set aside.

5. In the bowl with the dry cake ingredients, add the CBD-infused coconut oil and combine with the dry ingredients until distributed evenly. Add the water to the aquafaba, stir, and then add to the dry ingredients while mixing. The batter should be dough-like.

6. Spread the batter into the baking pan and arrange the apples on top into a design or neat rows for visual appeal.

7. Bake for 35 minutes or until the apples are a little brown and a toothpick comes out clean from the center. Remove from the oven and allow to cool on the countertop.

8. Slice the cake into as many servings as you wish. Enjoy immediately or store in a closed container in the refrigerator for up to a week. The cake slices can be warmed again or served cold.

Lemon Poppyseed Fruit Salad

Need a spectacular dish for a picnic or potluck? You can't go wrong with this CBD-infused fruit salad! Nutritious and easy to make any time.

Makes several servings

5 cups (1kg) or more of cut fruit and berries of your choice
1 cup (160g) shelled hemp seeds
1 tbsp (15ml) seltzer water
2 tbsp (30ml) CBD-infused MCT oil (page 18)
¼ cup (60ml) lemon juice
1 tsp (1g) grated lemon zest
⅓ cup (80ml) honey
1 tbsp (8g) poppy seeds

1. Put the cut, mixed fruit in a large salad bowl or other large serving bowl.

2. To a blender, add the hemp seeds, seltzer water, CBD oil, lemon juice, lemon zest, and honey. Blend until smooth and creamy. Pour into a bowl. Add the poppy seeds and stir.

3. Pour the mixture over the cut fruit and toss to combine. Serve immediately. Serve within one day for best flavor; hemp seeds have less pleasant flavor after a day or more.

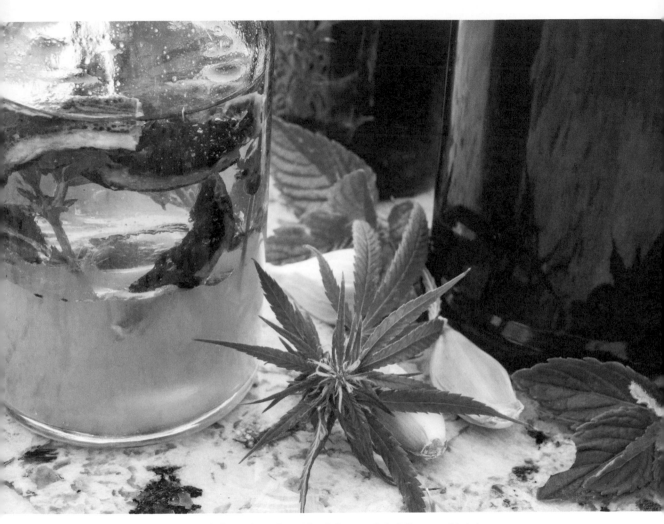

Yuzu Ginger Salad Dressing (left) and *Sicilian Blood Orange Salad Dressing* (right)

The Savory

Salad dressing is an outstanding way to enjoy CBD because it will infuse into many different kinds of oils. If you are using whole flower and leaf infusions, even better! The herbal flavor of the cannabis marries perfectly with the other flavors in the dressings here.

Yuzu Ginger Salad Dressing

Makes 1 cup (240ml) dressing

⅔ cup (160ml) yuzu juice
1 large thumb-sized piece fresh ginger, peeled
2 tbsp (30ml) honey
1 tsp (6g) sea salt
1 tsp (2g) white pepper
⅓ cup (80ml) CBD-infused rice bran oil (page 20)

1. Prepare a salad dressing bottle or other container (glass only) to store and serve the salad dressing.
2. Put all of the ingredients in a blender. Blend until smooth. Transfer to the final container for serving and storage.
3. Shake the dressing to combine thoroughly before using. Keep refrigerated and use within one week.

Sicilian Blood Orange Salad Dressing

Makes 1 cup (240ml) dressing

½ cup (120ml) fresh-squeezed blood orange juice
3 tbsp (45ml) distilled white vinegar
1 tsp (1g) grated blood orange zest
1 large garlic clove
1 tsp (6g) sea salt
1 tsp (2g) cracked black pepper
⅓ cup (80ml) CBD-infused olive oil (page 22)
⅓ cup (8g) fresh basil

1. Prepare a salad dressing bottle or other container (glass only) to store and serve the salad dressing.
2. Put all of the ingredients, except for the basil, in a blender. Blend until smooth. Add the basil to the blender to chop it into shreds, but do not blend smooth.
3. Transfer to the final container for serving and storage. Shake the dressing to combine thoroughly before using. Keep refrigerated and use within one week.

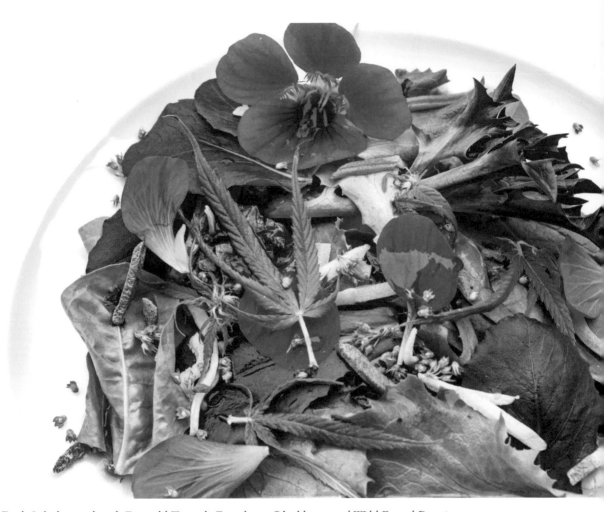

Fresh Salad topped with Emerald Triangle Farmhouse Blackberry and Wild Fennel Dressing

Emerald Triangle Farmhouse Blackberry and Wild Fennel Salad Dressing

Makes 1 cup (240ml) dressing

1 heaping cup (150g) fresh blackberries

⅓ cup (80ml) distilled white vinegar

1 large garlic clove

1 tsp (6g) sea salt

1 tsp (2g) cracked green peppercorn

3 tbsp (45ml) CBD-infused MCT oil (page 18)

¼ cup (60ml) hemp seed oil

¼ cup (4g) fresh fennel fronds

1. Prepare a salad dressing bottle or other container (glass only) to store and serve the salad dressing.
2. Put all the ingredients, except for the fennel fronds, in a blender. Blend until smooth. Add the fennel fronds to the blender to chop them into shreds, but do not blend smooth.
3. Transfer to the final container for serving and storage. Shake the dressing to combine thoroughly before using. Keep refrigerated and use within one week.

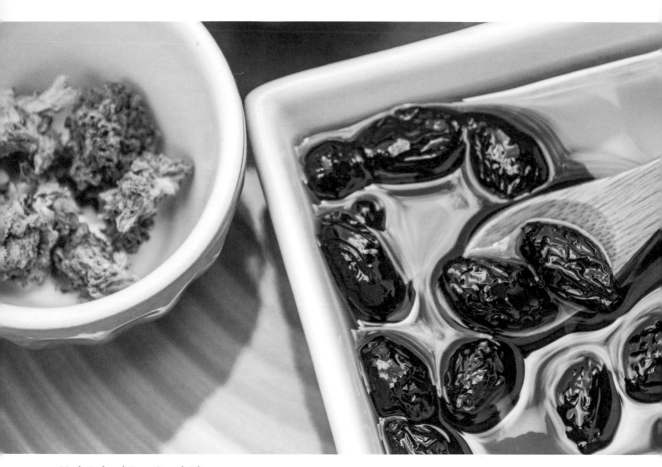

Herb-Infused Dry-Cured Olives

Herb-Infused Dry-Cured Olives

I began dry-curing my own olives several years ago in the San Francisco Bay area, where olive trees grow everywhere as an invasive species. Removing these fruits from the environment is not only good for the native flora, but there are also so many ways to enjoy them! My favorite way is dry-cured and then infused with herbs and high-quality CBD cannabis-infused olive oil. Dry cured wild olives are quite expensive in specialty supermarkets so if you live in an area where these trees are aplenty, preparing your own is a satisfying way to enjoy this exquisite gourmet treat.

If you don't live in an area where olive trees grow in abundance, don't fret—you can purchase dry-cured olives and infuse them with herbs and CBD. These olives should come in a package or jar with no additional oil added to them as shown here.

Dry-cured olives will always be black olives. If you are going to dry cure your own olives, pick them when they are black and fully ripe for the best flavor.

The great thing about having a jar of these on hand at all times is that they are a delicious and fast way to enjoy a dose of CBD anytime—just eat them straight from the jar! Keep the jar from moisture and light in a cool cabinet and they will last up to a year in storage.

The oil these olives are stored in will become quite flavorful with pronounced olive and herbal flavors and can be used to make delicious salad dressings or even bread dips.

If you are starting with raw, freshly picked black olives, the recipe to cure them is a simple one. If you are starting with olives that have already been dry-cured, you may skip this step and go right to the herbal infusion.

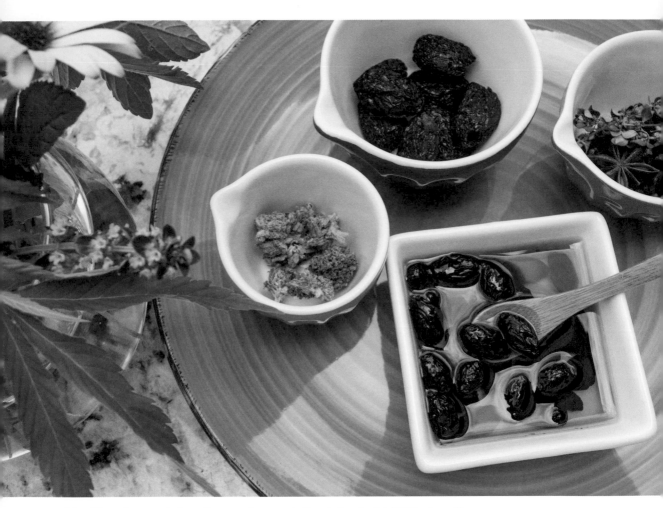

(Top: Plain dry-cured olives Bottom: dry-cured olives infused with CBD olive oil)

Dry-Curing Fresh Black Olives

1 muslin, cotton, or hemp drawstring bag

Kosher or sea salt, enough to fully cover the olives in the bag with room to spare

Fresh black olives, washed and dried completely

1. Pour a thick layer of salt at the bottom of the bag and then add a single layer of olives on top of it. Cover the olives with salt until completely buried. Add another single layer of olives and cover those until completely buried. Continue until all the olives have been layered in salt and bury the last layer of olives in an extra layer of salt.

2. Tie the bag together and hang it in a dry area for 3 to 4 weeks. The salt will draw out the moisture and most of the bitter compounds from the olives while salting them for preservation. During this drying period, it may be necessary to add more salt if the bag is too moist. The bag should remain mostly dry on the outside.

3. After the curing and drying process is over, open the bag and pour the salt and olives into a bowl. Remove the olives from the salt and put them in a separate container. The olives should be dry and wrinkled. Taste one. It should taste salty and nutty. Black olives are naturally slightly bitter. If the olives are dry and wrinkled, they are ready for the next step. If they are still moist, bury them in fresh salt again for another week—this should solve any additional moisture issues. The olives should be chewy but dry before you move on to the infusion process.

CBD Herbal Infusion and Oil Cure

There are a number of ways to infuse the olives with flavors and CBD. Some methods, such as whole CBD flowers, will have pronounced cannabis flavors. This can be surprisingly good with olives and other herbal flavors! Olives are certainly one food that can hold their own with stronger cannabis flavors. If you would prefer a lighter cannabis flavor, or no cannabis flavor at all, you will want to oil cure these olives in CBD-infused olive oil that has been prepared with either CBD resin or hashish with very little to no flavor. (See page 22 for preparing CBD-infused olive oil.)

Infuse and Cure with Whole CBD Flowers and Spices

This process requires approximately 1 month of shelf curing time. To decarboxylate your CBD flowers, process the oil and flowers in a canning jar and hot-water bath as described on page 22.

This recipe calls for dried whole spices and herbs. Use *only* spices and herbs that are dry; fresh or moist herbs will introduce moisture, which can spoil the oil cure. Some ideas for whole spices are black peppercorns, white peppercorns, thyme, basil, allspice, dried garlic, dried onion, dried red pepper, etc. Be as creative as you like and use a generous amount of spices.

1. In a clean jar, add the olives and herbs by creating layers of olives buried in layers of herbs. Pack tightly.
2. Pour the CBD-infused olive oil over the olives and herbs. Make sure the oil covers them completely and leave a little space at the top of the jar (½ inch [13mm]). Affix the lid and place them in a cool, dark cabinet or other area to rest and infuse for at least a month. These olives are even better when allowed to infuse for three months!

Dried, salt-cured black olives

Dried whole spices and herbs, as discussed

1 jar CBD flowers decarbed in CBD-infused olive oil in a canning bath as described on page 22

When the olives are ready, they can be served individually from the jar with the herbs and the oil can be used as a base for salad dressings or even bread dips. Make sure that enough oil remains in the jar to fully cover the olives and herbs that remain. Add more CBD-infused olive oil if necessary. Use within one year for the best flavor and CBD benefits.

Garlic Rosemary Popcorn

A great popcorn recipe for movie night at home! If you love the flavor of garlic and rosemary together, you will love this CBD-infused olive oil recipe.

Makes several servings

1 tbsp + 1 tsp (20ml) CBD-infused olive oil (page 22)
1 large garlic clove, shredded or chopped
¼ cup (90g) or more popcorn kernels
1 tbsp (3g) fresh rosemary leaves, chopped
1 tsp (6g) sea salt

1. In a pan on the stove, add the CBD oil and the garlic and combine to evenly coat the pan. Add the popcorn kernels and then sprinkle the rosemary and salt on top. Cover the pan.
2. Turn the heat to medium-high and pop the popcorn. Serve immediately.

Levantine Bread

Levantine breads are flat loaves typical of the cuisine of the Levant. The traditional recipes for these breads are rich in olive oil and herbal flavors, which makes them a great way to enjoy the benefits of CBD-infused olive oils in a savory dish. This loaf recipe is both gluten-free and big-eight allergen-free, which makes it great for many occasions and guests.

You can add many seasonings and toppings to these loaves, and creating your own blends is part of the fun! Za'atar is one of the most popular, but seasonings such as curry spice or hot spice blends like Harissa make excellent toppings as well as roasted onions, fennel, and garlic. This is delicious plain or with hummus or other dips.

Makes 4 (6- to 8-inch) loaves

1. In a bowl, add all of the za'atar topping ingredients and combine thoroughly. Note that you should only use whole hemp seeds; do not use shelled hemp seeds. Omit if this ingredient is not available or substitute with sesame. Set this aside to infuse while you prepare the loaves.
2. In another bowl, add all of the dry loaf ingredients and combine thoroughly. Add the olive oil and work it evenly through the dry ingredients. Slowly add the seltzer water and work this into the mixture. Continue to mix until the ingredients come together and you can knead into a ball. Once the ingredients are kneaded into a clean, smooth ball, put it back in the bowl, cover, and refrigerate for 15 minutes.
3. Roll the dough into 2 to 4 balls, depending on how big you want your loaves to be. Place one of the balls between two pieces of parchment paper and roll into a round loaf using a rolling pin. Do this for each of the loaves.
4. In a flat pan, roti pan, or tortilla pan on the stove, add a little olive oil and spread it around the pan to create a slick surface. Turn the burner

Za'atar topping ingredients:

1 tsp (2g) cumin
1 tsp (1g) minced dried onion
½ tsp (2g) garlic powder
1 tsp (2g) sumac
½ tsp (3g) sea salt
½ tsp (1g) allspice
¼ tsp (0.5g) cracked black pepper
¼ tsp (0.5g) dried red pepper
1 medium-sized CBD cannabis leaf, finely chopped
1 tbsp (5g) fresh lemon or regular thyme, finely chopped and packed
1 tbsp (5g) fresh oregano, finely chopped and packed
1 tbsp (5g) fresh marjoram, finely chopped and packed
2 tsp (4g) fresh fennel flowers (substitute with chopped fennel fronds if necessary), finely chopped and packed
1 tbsp (15ml) or a little more CBD-infused olive oil (page 22)
Whole toasted hemp seeds to sprinkle

Loaf Ingredients:

- 1 cup (180g) sweet brown rice flour
- ½ cup (80g) millet flour
- 2 tbsp (15g) mung dal flour
- 2 tbsp (18g) arrowroot flour
- ½ tsp (3g) sea salt
- 1 tbsp (15ml) olive oil
- ½ cup + 1 tbsp (135ml) seltzer water (use a little more if necessary throughout the dough kneading and resting process)

to medium-high heat and allow the pan to heat to the point that the oil begins to sizzle a bit.

5. Peel one of the loaves from the parchment paper and immediately add to the pan. Allow the loaf to cook in the pan until it starts to bubble and puff, about 2 minutes. Reduce the heat to medium. Flip the loaf and allow it to cook for another 1 to 2 minutes.

6. After cooking each of the loaves, transfer to a plate using a spatula. Prepare the oven by preheating to broil. Place each of the loaves next to each other on a baking sheet.

7. Stir the za'atar topping and spoon it evenly over each of the loaves. Add any other additional topping that you enjoy, such as sliced fennel bulbs. Put them in the oven and broil for about 3 minutes, until sizzling on top. Remove from the oven and serve hot!

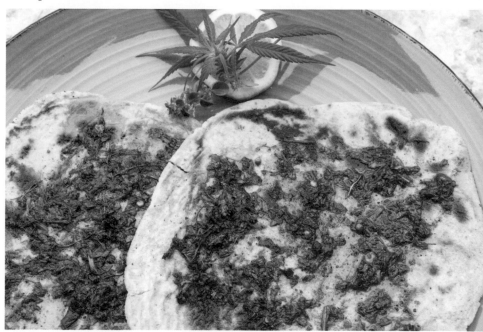

Jerk Roasted Pumpkin Seeds

One of my personal favorites for movie night at home! Don't throw away your pumpkin or squash seeds; save them (they can be frozen if you can't make this recipe right away) to make this delicious CBD-infused snack. If you love hot and spicy, you will love this, but if you would like to back off some of the heat, use less of the habanero pepper.

Makes several servings

1. Preheat the oven to 360° F (182° C). Line a baking sheet with parchment paper and set aside.
2. Scrape the seeds from the pumpkin or squash, clean the strings and fibers out of the seeds, but do not wash the seeds so that the flavor is retained.
3. In a bowl, combine all the seasoning ingredients, including the CBD oil. Add this to the bowl with the pumpkin or squash seeds and toss to combine thoroughly.
4. Spread the seasoned seeds in one layer on the baking sheet lined with parchment paper. Roast in the oven for 10 to 15 minutes or until a little brown. Remove from the oven. These can be served immediately, or they will store for a week in an airtight container.

Seeds scraped from 1 or 2 fresh pumpkins or squash, unwashed
1 tbsp (3g) fresh thyme OR lemon thyme
1 tbsp (3g) fresh parsley
1 fresh habanero pepper, chopped, seeds removed
1 tsp (2g) allspice
1 tsp (2g) garlic powder
1 tsp (2g) onion powder
1½ tsp (8g) sea salt
½ tsp (1g) cracked black pepper
1 tbsp (15ml) lemon juice
1–2 tbsp (15ml–30ml) CBD-infused coconut oil, melted

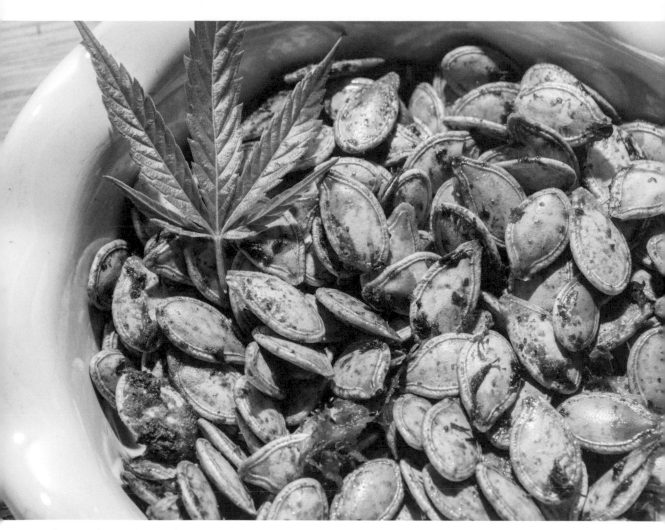

Jerk Roasted Pumpkin Seeds

RESOURCES

The most comprehensive information resource about CBD that I have found has been Project CBD (projectcbd.org), and I recommend this site as a starting point for you to educate yourself and your family about CBD.

Scents of Earth https://scents-of-earth.com/ is a favorite source for purchasing rare resins and herbs.

Richter Herbs https://www.richters.com/ has every aromatic plant and seed that you will ever need. If you are ready to start an aromatic plant garden, check out this store first.

Persian Basket https://persianbasket.com/ is where I purchase all of my saffron and other exotic Middle Eastern spices and kitchen accessories.

Amazon https://www.amazon.com Amazon almost always has hard-to-find and quality ingredients in stock.

Monterey Bay Spice Company https://www.herbco.com carries many of the herbs I use, especially the less-well-known and hard to find herbs like soapwort.

Mountain Rose Herbs https://www.mountainroseherbs.com/ is a well-respected herbal apothecary and spa supply store. Highly recommended.

Banyan Botanicals https://www.banyanbotanicals.com carries very high quality, food-grade boswellia (frankincense) and other herbs.

Better Bee https://www.betterbee.com/ is my trusted resource for reasonably priced and high-quality bayberry and beeswax

ABOUT THE AUTHOR

I'm an author, a certified allergy chef (certified in both Allertrain and ServSafe Allergens), a home herbalist for more than twenty-five years—and as many years as an experienced forager of wild food, flowers, and herbs—a visual artist, and webmaster. Today I am a coastal resident of Del Norte County, California, which is the tip of the "Emerald Triangle" in Northern California. I live with my geeky husband and sassy parrot. I like to garden, collect driftwood and agates, and spend much of my time in my kitchen formulating new spa and culinary creations.

I am also a survivor of multiple autoimmune disease and an anaphylactic who carries Epipens for life-threatening food and environmental allergies. In 2011, I was diagnosed with multiple autoimmune diseases and a rare autoimmune condition known as Orbital Pseudotumor and Sarcoidosis. I received treatment for several years at Stanford Hospital including radiation and immune therapy. I am forever grateful for the brilliant doctors who saved my life.

I learned my toughest life lesson when I was fighting for my life and my eyesight: my immune system makes the rules for me—I don't get a choice. Autoimmune disease and adult anaphylactic allergies are incurable, and I will have these for the rest of my life. The feeling of the loss of control—the fact that I had no vote or voice in the decisions my immune system was making for me—was devastating. I'm still learning to cope with this, even as I write this new book.

Pain management is a special interest of mine because it's been a coping mechanism for me—an aspect of my health that I can control, and why I am an advocate for cannabis. Chronic pain is a debilitating condition but also a subjective and individual experience. As a patient advocate, I think patients should be trusted and believed. I understand what it's like to walk down that path of pharmaceutical pain management because I have been there; I have experienced the loss of control and the inevitable outcome of these drugs when they eventually lose their effectiveness after long-term use. Learning to manage my own chronic pain with the help of cannabis and herbs in the privacy of my home has been my greatest gift to myself. And with my books, I hope that it is a gift I am able to share with many people.

If I get to choose the legacy I leave in this life, it will be the number of people I have led away from pharmaceutical pain pills who suffer from chronic pain like I do—reclaiming our liberty to self-manage pain in the privacy of our homes with gentle herbs like cannabis. I am passionate about serving my autoimmune and allergy community and everyone who suffers chronic pain. I hope that you will find comfort and joy through my writings, recipes, and handmade goods!

—Sandra Hinchliffe

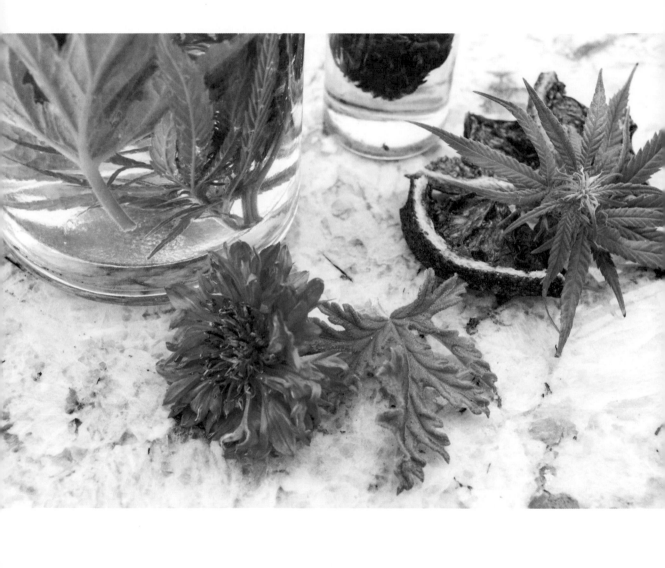

INDEX

Mood Therapy Tincture, 100
Quick Relief Tincture, 97
"Roll Your Own" Pain Pills, 103–105
Sun Salute Massage Oil, 65–67
Fresh Pear Bhang, 111

G

Garlic Rosemary Popcorn, 131
geranium
    Deep Relief Massage Honey, 68–69
    Farmer's Salve, 49–51
    Minty Chocolate Lip Balm, 53–54
ginger
    Ginger and Turmeric Hemp Smoothie, 85
    Quick Relief Tincture, 97
    Revitalizing Dessert Soup, 93
    Spiced Lime Moringa Soup, 95
    Super Pain Balm, 61–62
    Winter Blues Herbal Broth, 96
    Yuzu Ginger Salad Dressing, 123
Ginger and Turmeric Hemp Smoothie, 85
goji berry
    Maiden Elixir, 88
Golden Goat, 5
Gooey Brownie Pie, 118
green peppercorn
    Emerald Triangle Farmhouse Blackberry and
        Wild Fennel Salad Dressing, 125
Gupta, Sanjay, 11

H

habanero pepper
    Jerk Roasted Pumpkin Seeds, 134
Harlequin, 5

Harle-Tsu, 5
hemp, 5
hemp seed oil
    Aromatic Herbal Soap, 73–75
    Emerald Triangle Farmhouse Blackberry and
        Wild Fennel Salad Dressing, 125
hemp seeds
    Ginger and Turmeric Hemp Smoothie, 85
    Lemon Poppyseed Fruit Salad, 121
    Levantine Bread, 132
herbal bath bombs
    Fragrant Herbal Bath Bombs, 77–78
Herbal Pills for What Ails You, 106–107
herbal soap
    Aromatic Herbal Soap, 73–75
herbal supplement market, 7–9
Herbes de Provence, 96
herbs, alternative, 37
high, 2, 11, 13–15
honey
    Deep Relief Massage Honey, 68–69
    Ginger and Turmeric Hemp Smoothie, 85
    Lemon Mint Fever Frosty, 81
    Lemon Poppyseed Fruit Salad, 121
    Yuzu Ginger Salad Dressing, 123
hot pepper
    Whipped Chocolate Body Butter, 55–56

I

infusions
    aromatic, 46–47
    for beverage, 35
    for broth, 35
    dry salt and soda, 47

T

terpene infusion, 47

test results, 9

Thai peppers

    Spiced Lime Moringa Soup, 95

THC (tetrahydrocannabinol), 1

THC ratio, 10–13

thyme, 88

    Farmer's Salve, 49–51

    Jerk Roasted Pumpkin Seeds, 134

    Levantine Bread, 132

tincture, 29–34

    Crone Elixir, 88

    Detox Tincture, 101

    Effervescent Magnesium Cocktails, 87–88

    Mood Therapy Tincture, 100

    Quick Relief Tincture, 97

    Sleepy-Time Tincture, 99

    Winter Blues Herbal Broth, 96

tomatoes

    Winter Blues Herbal Broth, 96

Turkish rose

    Ave Maria Balm, 63–64

turmeric

    Ginger and Turmeric Hemp Smoothie, 85

    Sleepy-Time Tincture, 99

    Super Pain Balm, 61–62

V

vanilla bean

    Deep Relief Massage Honey, 68–69

    Whipped Chocolate Body Butter, 55–56

vessel, 42–46

W

water-oil infusion, 46

Whipped Chocolate Body Butter, 55–56

white peppercorn

    Spiced Lime Moringa Soup, 95

white pine resin

    Forest Elixir, 91

whole-plant material, 17

Wild Emerald Herbs Salve, 51–52

Winter Blues Herbal Broth, 96

Y

Yuzu Ginger Salad Dressing, 123

Z

za'atar topping, 132

THE CANNABIS SPA AT HOME

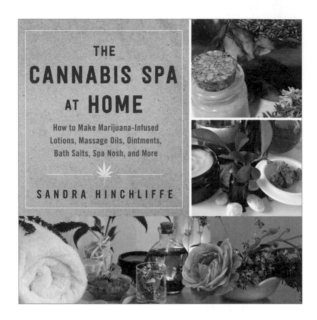

Hardcover ISBN: 978-1-63450-230-6
Paperback ISBN: 978-1-5107-4088-4

The Cannabis Spa at Home contains more than seventy-five cannabis spa recipes free of preservatives and major allergens that can be prepared in the home kitchen or professional spa with wholesome herbal ingredients.

HIGH TEA

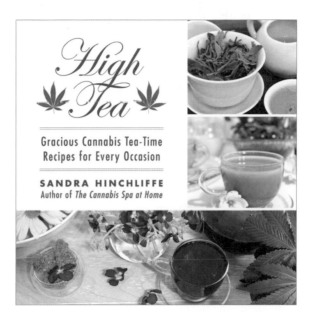

Hardcover ISBN: 978-1-5107-1757-2

With *High Tea*, author Sandra Hinchliffe writes a totally new chapter in tea culture and the culinary art of cannabis cuisine. Teas, tisanes, broths, and bhangs are all exquisite ways to infuse marijuana for medicine or pleasure.

With more than seventy-five recipes using a fascinating array of the finest teas, herbs, and ingredients, High Tea will show you how to create sensational flavors, select moods, and serve all the good vibrations the cannabis plant has to offer.

CONVERSION CHARTS

Metric and Imperial Conversions

(These conversions are rounded for convenience)

Ingredient	Cups/ Tablespoons/ Teaspoons	Ounces	Grams/ Milliliters
Fruit, dried	1 cup	4 ounces	120 grams
Fruits or veggies, chopped	1 cup	5 to 7 ounces	145 to 200 grams
Fruits or veggies, puréed	1 cup	8.5 ounces	245 grams
Honey, maple syrup, or corn syrup	1 tablespoon	0.75 ounce	20 grams (15 milliliters)
Liquids: cream, milk, water, or juice	1 cup	8 fluid ounces	240 milliliters
Salt	1 teaspoon	0.2 ounces	6 grams
Spices: cinnamon, cloves, ginger, or nutmeg (ground)	1 teaspoon	0.2 ounce	5 milliliters (2 grams)
Sugar, brown, firmly packed	1 cup	7 ounces	200 grams
Sugar, white	1 cup/ 1 tablespoon	7 ounces/0.5 ounce	200 grams/12.5 grams
Vanilla extract	1 teaspoon	0.2 ounce	4 grams (5 milliliters)

Liquids

8 fluid ounces = 1 cup = ½ pint
16 fluid ounces = 2 cups = 1 pint
32 fluid ounces = 4 cups = 1 quart
128 fluid ounces = 16 cups = 1 gallon